Ross W. Halpin

Jewish Doctors and the Holocaust

Ross W. Halpin

Jewish Doctors and the Holocaust

The Anatomy of Survival in Auschwitz

DE GRUYTER
OLDENBOURG   MAGNES

ISBN 978-3-11-059604-5
e-ISBN (PDF) 978-3-11-059821-6
e-ISBN (EPUB) 978-3-11-059375-4

Library of Congress Control Number: 2018955640

Bibliographic information published by the Deutsche Nationalbibliothek
The Deutsche Nationalbibliothek lists this publication in the Deutsche Nationalbibliografie;
detailed bibliographic data are available in the Internet at http://dnb.dnb.de.

© 2018 Walter de Gruyter GmbH, Berlin/Boston & Hebrew University Magnes Press, Jerusalem
Editing: Marie-Louise Bethune
Typesetting: Integra Software Services Pvt. Ltd.
Printing and binding: CPI books GmbH, Leck
Cover image: The Syringe: An execution by needle Sketch by David Olere. Courtesy of Mr Serge
Klarsfeld.

www.degruyter.com

There are places that will scream forever
    Stanislaw Ryniak (First prisoner of Auschwitz No. 31)

                    'If it be but a world of agony.' –
                    'Whence camest thou? and whither goest thou?
                    How did thy course begin?' I said, 'and why?

                    'Mine eyes are sick of this perpetual flow
                    Of people, and my heart sick of one sad thought –
                    Speak!' – 'Whence I am, I partly seem to know,

                    'And how and by what paths I have been brought
                    To this dread pass, methinks even thou mays guess; –
                    Why this should be, my mind can compass not;

            The Triumph of Life

                    Percy Bysshe Shelley

In Memory

Dr Sima Vaisman

Dr Gisella Perl

Dr Louis Micheels

and

all Jewish doctors who survived Auschwitz
and those who paid the ultimate price

Harm befalls a wicked messenger
A faithful courier brings healing
Proverbs 13:17

To Rosie

Foreword

Etienne Lepicard

This book is an unusual work among Holocaust scholarship. It asks an unusual research question – How do people survive Auschwitz? It uses unusual sources – mostly memoirs of survivors, quite often and justly considered as problematic by historians. It builds an unusual tool to answer its question – a bio-psychosocial model for survival assessment. While it focuses on the fate of a few Jewish doctors who survived Auschwitz, it results in broader openings able to meet the quest of every one.

How to describe what the Jewish doctors went through when there are almost no sources remaining? How can one rely on what has been written after the war, when we know how much emotions were involved in that writing? These are some of the issues every researcher about the Holocaust has to cope with, notwithstanding his own feelings. Ross Halpin in this beautifully written book goes through them in a wonderful manner, not hesitating from time to time to share with us part of his own personal journey through research. And still he tells us a story well grounded into current scholarship on the Holocaust.

In this sense, the author's description of Auschwitz' medical world is an illuminating and brilliant synthesis and his final chapter, 'Anatomy of survival,' a masterpiece, where one can see his own contribution to research at its best. However, what I found much impressive is the way Halpin knew how to 'listen' to his sources – memoirs written immediately after the war or later on, not only to read them but to make them speak to him and tell an almost unutterable story. As well, he knew how to meet survivors' family and again listen to them, this time to hear their quest for life illuminating his own quest: 'I suddenly realized that I was not researching death. Instead I was examining the quest for life.'

Etienne Lepicard (MD, PhD), Bet Hagat and the Israeli National Council for Bioethics, Jerusalem

https://doi.org/10.1515/9783110598216-201

Preface

I did not die, and I was not alive;
think for yourself, if you have any wit,
what I became, deprived of life and death.
Dante Alighieri (1995)

It is 7 am, in early December 2010 and the Polish winter is bitterly cold. Every morning for the past 10 days Danuta, the owner of the B&B where I am staying, has driven me to Auschwitz Concentration Camp. We drive in silence because she does not speak or understand English and I know few words in Polish. The streets of Oświęcim are mostly deserted. The intense silence helps me to absorb my surroundings as we approach the camp. Very fine snowflakes touch the windscreen and disappear while a layer of mist hangs softly over the grounds of the camp. Although daylight has come, there is a terrible darkness about the camp, and I always feel the same sense of foreboding. My fear is that on this occasion I will not be able to go inside.

'Dziękuę,' I say in thanks to Danuta and she replies 'Do zobaczonia o czwartej,' indicating she will return at four o'clock to pick me up as usual after yet another day of research. I walk towards the gates and pass under the infamous sign, Arbeit Macht Frei. On the left is the SS guard room. Entering the camp, I pass the area to the right where the prisoner band played as inmates, most half dead, left for and returned from hard labour. The footsteps of a staff member walking on the cobblestones break the silence. I arrive outside block 14 and turn right into a street that is lined with poplars and occupied by rows and rows of blocks. Blocks 4, 5, 6 and 7 on my left and 16, 17 and 18 on my right are now exhibition centers, but I cannot forget that they were living quarters and death chambers for prisoners. The specter of death is they omnipresent.

I am desperately cold and alone yet I can sense the ghostly shadows of the dead around me. Skeletal filthy bodies with grotesque frozen faces are heaped outside the entrance to the blocks. Others have been loaded into barrows pushed or drawn by emaciated fellow prisoners. I cannot imagine another place like it on earth. It is literally a graveyard on which ashes from the chimneys have been spread. Visitors are walking on the dead.

Each block had its own history, but death had been common to them all. The prisoners had been penned in like animals waiting for slaughter. Before death had come suffering, pain, fear, and most certainly the loss of hope. What do they say? 'Hope is the last to die.' I continued until I reached the hospital blocks, 19, 20 and 21 on the right and, finally, on the left: Block 10, my destination. The doors were locked and the windows shuttered. This block was unique. It personified

https://doi.org/10.1515/9783110598216-202

evil. It was here that grotesque human medical experiments had been performed on young Jewish women. Most of the women had died; those who did survive were rendered sterile.

It was during my visits to Block 10 to conduct research on the Holocaust and Nazi medicine (Halpin 2011) that I discovered two startling facts which germinated into the idea of writing this book: firstly, that Jewish doctors worked, most against their will, with the Nazi doctors; secondly, that Jewish doctors treated prisoner patients in the hospitals and infirmaries. It didn't make sense to me that an extermination camp should have its own medical system, with hospitals, infirmaries and clinics, supposedly for treating and caring for prisoners. On closer investigation I discovered that following heavy losses to the Russians in early 1942, Germany needed a workforce; while they were still alive and able to work, prisoners in the concentration camps could supply this labor. Thus, the hospitals and infirmaries in the death camp and the Jewish doctors who worked in them played an important role in the life of the camp and involuntarily and unknowingly contributed to Germany's war effort.

This was intriguing. I wanted to understand why Jewish doctors in Auschwitz became important to the SS. I had many questions, but despite my best efforts, I could not find answers. How many Jewish doctors worked in Auschwitz? Were they recognized as doctors or orderlies? Were some collaborators? Did they enjoy special privileges? What were their working conditions? What ethical, moral and religious dilemmas did they face? Or were the doctor's decisions and actions influenced more by the human condition and under the circumstances of being faced by 'choicelesss choices' than by ethical dilemmas? I decided to follow the journey of this specific group of prisoners from their entry into the camp and track their tortuous passage through the system. I wanted to learn about their experiences and find out how long they survived.

My first task was to examine historical sources; my next to consult memoirs of survivors and oral testimonies. A number of memoirs were available, but there was practically no reliable historical material to be found and no evidence of research into the experience and fate of Jewish doctors held captive in Nazi concentration and labor camps. I searched the archives at Auschwitz for medical and camp records which might document the activities of Jewish doctors and hopefully provide a window into the life of Jewish doctors in Auschwitz. Alas, there was very little data available, certainly insufficient to produce a comprehensive and meaningful history. Before their flight from the camp on 18th January 1945, the SS destroyed as much official documentation as possible, including material I desperately needed. The Jewish doctors had been rendered invisible in documented history thereby allowing them to become a 'forgotten' group.

I decided to return to Warsaw. I boarded the train frustrated with my lack of success at finding 'worthwhile' information at Auschwitz and mulled over what to do next. Was it worth continuing this line of investigation or should I move on to other areas of interest regarding the Holocaust and medicine? Unbeknownst to me, the documents on my lap would point me in an entirely different and more significant direction. As I began reading the material I had gathered over the past eight days, I found that approximately forty-eight of the seventy Jewish doctors I had researched survived Auschwitz. On collating their dates of arrival at the camp and the date of arrival of those who survived into the DP (Displaced Persons) camps after the War, I found that these Jewish doctors had survived an average of 20 months. This was astounding. I knew from previous research that the average life span of Jewish prisoners thrown into slave labor was twelve weeks while many survived for only twenty-one days. In a death camp where every Jewish prisoner was under a death sentence and the vast majority perished, how did the doctor prisoner survive nearly ten times as long as the ordinary prisoner?

The subject of Jewish doctors and their role in concentration, labor and extermination camps during the Holocaust has been a marginalized theme in Holocaust research. Even more marginalized has been the epic and extraordinary struggle to survive of a small group of doctors from Auschwitz. The story I have uncovered after five years of research into the survival of Jewish doctors during the Holocaust is one of courage, altruism, sacrifice and inspiration. In a sea of evil these doctors maintained their dignity and displayed humanity towards their fellow human beings, be they Jews or non-Jews. It is also a human story of doctors who were ordinary people with similar strengths and weaknesses that led them to act against religious, moral, ethical and personal standards in order to survive. Under conditions of extreme adversity, in which there was no relief from suffering and there appeared to be no escape from death, most prisoners soon fell into a state of despair, lost all hope and died within a short time, often within days of entering the camp. According to Primo Levi (1988 , 90), these prisoners formed 'the backbone of the camp' which he called an 'anonymous mass.' They were referred to in Auschwitz as Muselmänner[1] and without the will to live starved themselves to death, were worked to death, beaten to death or executed because they were incapable of following orders. The survivors existed in a situation where there was a beginning but they could see no end, as though they were walking through a thick fog yet despite the seeming impossibility of escaping death, they refused to surrender and allow death to claim them. In making this statement I do not mean those who died or were murdered were lessor people. I

---

1 The concept of *Muselmänner* will be addressed more thoroughly in following chapters.

do not agree with Dwork, who argues that 'survival must be attributed to nothing more – or less – than luck and fortuitous circumstances', adding historians who propose survival was dependent on adaptive behavior or the will to live was she contends an 'act of failure or stupidity on the part of those who were murdered' (Dwork 1995 , 93). As Peter Suedfeld responded to which I agree and for which there is no basis her theory is unjust and unjustified by the example of the murder of 1.5 million innocent babies, infants and children.

The survivors did not have any extraordinary single powers or strengths. Instead, it was a set of circumstances and personal qualities that buoyed them and allowed these doctors, ordinary people, to survive extreme adversity.

Acknowledgements

This book was born from my previous and ongoing research into unscientific and unethical human medical experiments by Nazi SS doctors. The book has taken five years of exhaustive research regarding the work and survival of Jewish doctors in the death camps, in this case, Auschwitz extermination camp. The process has involved interviewing Holocaust survivors, relatives and friends of Jewish doctors who survived, many, many trips to Holocaust museums and research centres throughout the world and visits, sometimes for days and weeks, at camp sites such as Auschwitz. In addition, I have presented papers at and attended international conferences related to my subject.

Investigating the terrible acts committed by the SS doctors during human experiments on Jewish prisoners was emotionally and physically exhausting however the personal toll visited upon me during the research and writing of this book was indescribable. I needed people to assist me academically, intellectually and emotionally. That is, I needed support. To thank everybody who gave me that support is obviously impossible so I apologise. There are however individuals I must thank who without them I could not have finished the project.

Emeritus Professor Dr Konrad Kwiet who was my supervisor during my doctorate dissertation, my mentor and who I humbly call my colleague. He is a world renowned Holocaust historian and I consider myself extremely privileged to have been privy to his knowledge and experience. I thank Professor Garry Walter AM, Dr Etienne Lepicard and Dr Astrid Ley for their constructive remarks during the defence of my dissertation that contributed to the quality of my work. To Louise Marie Bethune, my editor and dear friend who has worked with me for the past ten years. Marie Louise knows that I could not have achieved what I have without her. I thank Anat Wollenberger, my Hebrew and Yiddish translator in Israel, who for the past ten years has worked with me at Yad Vashem. Without her dedication to my project and continual support it would have been impossible to complete my work. I must thank all of my translators and research assistants; Polish, Hungarian and German although I did learn to read the latter solely for my research.

I owe a debt to the relatives and friends of survivors: Dr Gisella Perl, Dr Louis Micheels and Dr Sima Vaisman for sharing memories and providing photos and documents but also welcoming me into their homes. I was privileged to personally interview many Auschwitz survivors including Mr Kalman Bar On, Helen "Zippy" Tichauer and Lotte Weiss.

I would like to thank Yad Vashem for awarding me the Archival Research Scholarship in 2011 and Mr Nick Politis AM a Sydney based businessman for financially assisting me in my research. I appreciate the support extended to me

https://doi.org/10.1515/9783110598216-203

particularly in respect to travelling grants by the Department of Biblical, Hebrew and Jewish Studies at Sydney University. With respect to the publication of the book I express my gratitude to the staff at the Hebrew University Magnes Press: Professor Avigdor Shinan, Director Jonathon Nadav, Celestina Levant and Ruhama Haleui and those at De Gruyter Oldenbourg, in particular Dr Julia Brauch, Acquisitions Editor Jewish Studies & History.

On a personal basis I need to thank four very important people who, over the past 18 years, have given me wonderful support: Dr Prem Naidoo, Associate Professor Raymond Garrick, Associate Professor Jonathon Stretch and Dr Wayne Reid. In addition, without the empathy and moral and intellectual support of my wonderful wife, Rosie, this book would not have seen the light of day. Rosie was also my French translator.

Finally, how can one survive an ordeal such as the one I have endured over the last ten years including the research into Nazi human experimentation without the support of a loving family. To Rosie, my wife, and Simone, Kath, Liz, Ross, Steve and your families I thank you and send you all my love. To my sister Lyn and her family and Sally, Linda and Matthew and your respective families. Thank you.

I hope this work will add to the body of knowledge of the history of the Holocaust particularly the history of Jewish doctors during this very dark period.

Contents

Introduction

Rejected by mankind, the condemned do not go
so far as to reject it in turn. Their faith in history
remains unshaken, and one may well wonder why.
They do not despair. The proof: they persist in
surviving – not only to survive, but to testify.
The victims elect to become witnesses.
Terence Des Pres (1976)

On 15 December 1943, Dr Kurt Grunwald, his wife Vilma and their two sons Michael and John arrived in Auschwitz after two insufferable days and nights on a cattle train from Theresienstadt ghetto. Threatened and attacked by savage dogs and brutal baton-wielding SS guards, they found themselves encircled by evil and chaos. On the ramp, the family was sent to the right, selected to go to the labor camp. Grunwald worked as a doctor in Birkenau,[2] where the panicked screams of children as they were thrown alive into the flames belching from the pits[3] was as inescapable as the smoke and the stench of burning flesh and bones that blew straight into his barracks. On 10 July 1944, Grunwald lost his wife, his son John and his 71year-old mother to the gas chambers. On the 26th October 1944, he was separated from and lost contact with his son Michael. Despite living and working in Birkenau, the most murderous and evil concentration camp on earth, despite seeing children and babies murdered and having to select Jews to die, and despite knowing his family except Michael had perished, Kurt Grunwald survived Auschwitz. He lived to eventually find Michael and migrate to the United States, where he continued to work as a doctor.

How did Grunwald survive Auschwitz? How did Grunwald 'rise' to a level of human forbearance that could withstand such overwhelming suffering? With the pain of such loss, what drove him to continue, day after day, working in a place of such deprivation, cruelty, suffering, and death? Did he have inherent unique qualities of emotional and mental strength? Did he rely on his faith? I will present a case and construct to argue that Grunwald's survival and the survival of a relatively small group of Jewish doctors was neither random, happenstance nor due to faith; it was the result of conscious and unconscious factors that, barring accidents, illness or execution, gave them the moral and emotional strength to cope with and survive extreme stress and adversity. Auschwitz was an unforgiving

---

2 See Appendix 1. P.191.
3 Fire pits were used when the gas chambers and ovens were working at full capacity or near full capacity and there was a backlog of trains waiting to arrive at the ramps.

https://doi.org/10.1515/9783110598216-001

place where every prisoner was sentenced to death – either immediately upon arrival or after suffering unimaginable cruelty and fear before they were relieved of their pain. Some, such as Grunwald, coped and survived for months. According to Kahana and others, when coping with extreme stress:

> The total life experience is disrupted... the new environment is extremely hostile and dangerous... opportunities to remove or act upon the stressor environment are severely limited; there is no predictable end to the experience; and the pain and the suffering associated with the experience appear to be meaningless and without rational explanation. (Kahana et al. 1988, 59)

Grunwald's survival is evidence of the depth and indestructibility of human endurance. As Marek Edelman (2016), a survivor of the Warsaw ghetto recalled, 'What matters most is life itself.'[4] The other significant factor that improved Grunwald and other doctors' chance of survival was the change in Nazi policy towards Jewish labour in the camps and the role assigned to Jewish doctors until early 1945. The catalyst for this change was the military defeat of Germany on the Eastern Front,[5] which not only disrupted Germany's strategies and ability to wage an effective war against the Allies, it also put an end to the National Socialists' political vision of establishing the utopian state.[6] In expectation of victory, the Nazis had anticipated amassing a slave labour force of over two million Russian POWs. Instead, their defeat was nothing short of catastrophic, resulting in a critical shortage of labour to meet the demands of the German domestic market and the war economy. Hitler's early successes were thwarted by Stalin's counter-offensive with the result that two million Russian soldiers captured by the Germans either starved or froze to death. By early 1942, approximately one-third

---

4 Marek Edelman died in 2009 and was the last surviving member of the Warsaw Ghetto Uprising in 1943. He was one of the few who escaped the ghetto. After the Second World War he remained in Poland, his home country, and became a doctor and cardiologist. He became active in the country's union movement (Edelman 2016).

5 Germany invaded the Soviet Union in the summer of 1941. It was a disastrous military operation for Germany leading to the loss of territory and over one million soldiers and approximately 25 million Soviet citizens died. In brief Germany lost the war for three main reasons. First the strategy of Blitzkrieg that was successful in the invasion of France did not work in the war against Russia. Second Russia was larger in territory in numbers than Germany including the power of a large army of partisans who were effective against the German foot soldiers. Third the German army was hopelessly ill equipped to cope with the winter conditions and Hitler ignored the advice of his generals and made disastrous decisions.

6 The perfect State was one free of Jewish blood and gypsies, homosexuals, criminals and the disabled. The goal of the National Socialist Party was to transform Germany into a *Volksgemeinschaft, a* community of racially pure Aryans.

of Germany's troops, over one million men, had been killed, lost or wounded.[7] The immediate effects of this defeat on both the domestic and war economies needed to be corrected or Germany's flagging fortunes would end in total capitulation. Germany was experiencing a critical shortage of labour and an immediate solution was required. As a result, the concentration and labour camps metaphorically became vehicles that would supply slave labour for the production of goods and services for both economies with priority given to the war economy. Auschwitz became the site of one of the largest industrial plants in Nazi-occupied territory in which over 400,000 Jewish slave labourers perished.

The new labour policy became even more demanding of the prisoners, often driven to the edge of their endurance as their hours of work were increased, the number of breaks reduced, and harsh and cruel punishment was inflicted. At the same time, the camp commandants were ordered to provide better treatment and care to sick and injured prisoners to enable them to return to work as quickly as possible. The orders even directed sick prisoners to do some type of work while in bed. It is difficult to imagine patients, in some cases twelve to a bunk, doing any work. The policy of increasing the labor force and ensuring Jews were fit enough to work took precedence over everything else, including the wholesale gassing of Jews. From early 1942 the urgency to turn Auschwitz into an industrial centre led to the uncontrolled and haphazard growth of the prison population. As a consequence, conditions became worse, the availability of food, clothing and bedding became critical and a matter of life and death and the spread and intensity of epidemics became uncontrollable. The chaos that followed tells the real story of why the SS were forced to assign Jewish doctors to the hospitals and infirmaries.

Auschwitz' prison population of approximately 1,000 inmates in 1940 grew to fluctuate between 28,000 and 156,000 during the period 1942 to 1944. From the very beginning, the SS doctors treated SS personnel, their families and the small group of prisoners, mainly Polish nationals, who arrived to help in the construction of the camp. By March 1941 the population was 10,100. During the early period, Jews were either selected for labour or were executed by shooting or in modified gas vans. Interestingly, Jewish doctors and other members of the intelligentsia were automatically selected for execution at that stage. In March 1941 Himmler ordered the camp to be expanded to hold 30,000 prisoners and later that year ordered the construction of Auschwitz-Birkenau, to house 100,000 prisoners. As the prisoner population grew, particularly the Jewish population,

---

7 According to M. Mazower (2009, 139), more German troops had frozen to death than died during the entire war on the British or American sides.

conditions in the camps worsened leading to epidemics and the death of tens of thousands of prisoners. Jews were considered sub-human. According to Giselle Perl, a Jewish doctor who worked in Birkenau:

> [There] was one latrine for thirty to thirty-two thousand women and we were permitted to use it only at certain hours of the day. We stood in line to get into this tiny building, knee-deep in human excrement. As we all suffered from dysentery, we could rarely wait until our turn came, and soiled our ragged clothes, which never came off our bodies ... The latrine consisted of a deep ditch with planks thrown across it at certain intervals. We squatted on these planks like birds perched on telegraph wire, so close together that we could not help soiling one another. (Perl 1948, 33)

The epidemics not only killed the inmates, the increasing death toll among the SS, their families and people in the villages and towns near the camps were causing the Nazis immediate concern. As a result, camps were quarantined, SS personnel were forbidden to enter particular areas, and SS doctors and non-Jewish doctors refused to treat Jewish and gypsy prisoners. Jewish prisoner doctors were identified at the railhead and assigned to work in the hospitals and infirmaries. One of the most ironic aspects of Auschwitz and Hitler's war against the Jews was the dependence of the SS on Jewish doctors to assist them. On the one hand, Jewish doctors were required to treat the prisoners to get them back to work where they would face an agonizing death from exhaustion, execution, beatings or other forms of punishment yet, on the other, they were ordered to select prisoners who were too ill to return to work for execution. Auschwitz was a slave labour camp and an industrialized murder machine of which the Jews were the main source and victims respectively.

Assignment to the hospitals and infirmaries gave Jewish doctors certain privileges, but they quickly learned the dark side of their positions. In addition to their fundamental responsibility to work in blocks treating patients, they were required to take part in *selections*[8] and barbaric medical experiments.

---

[8] The term *selection* is a euphemism for chosing a number of prisoners to be executed either by phenol, shooting or by gassing. These selections were carried out in the hospitals and infirmaries. The term *selection* was also applied at the train ramp and during roll calls. *Selections* in the hospitals took place to clear them of prisoners who could not return to work within a specific time, usually two weeks at the maximum. If a number of trains were arriving and a large number of fit but sick prisoners were expected *selections* would take place to ensure there were sufficient cots for these new patients. The SS doctors were ruthless in selecting prisoners for executions. The Jewish doctors who were responsible for the medical treatment of the prisoners were usually involved either directly (selecting) or indirectly (consulting) in *selections*. Over two thirds of the Jews sent to Auschwitz were sent to the gas chambers or shot or burnt to death upon reaching the camp through the *selection* method.

Due to a critical shortage of medications and medical supplies (bandages and plaster were as good as non-existent), doctors were also forced to choose who would receive what was available and who would go without, thus to some extent condemning certain patients to die. While they did benefit from the improved conditions that came with their status, life expectancy was always tenuous. A minority of Jewish doctors worked in research centres that provided better and more secure conditions, but the majority of doctors worked in Birkenau and the sub-labour camps where there was no respite from inhumanity and death. For an average of twenty months they were witness to human suffering and deprivation and to extreme acts of evil and wickedness. In addition, they were themselves subject to beatings and torture and under the constant threat of death.

Initially I struggled to understand how these doctors had survived physically, emotionally and psychologically against what seemed insurmountable odds. There had to be an explanation and it would have to be found in what these doctors had said and through their actions.

Over five years I examined the lives of 32 Jewish doctors who survived Auschwitz. To any who might question the significance of research on such a relatively small sample, my response is twofold: First, very few doctors survived Auschwitz, and even fewer wrote memoirs or gave testimonies. Second, even if only one doctor had survived and was able to bear witness to the conditions and provide a window into how it was possible to survive as a doctor in that camp, that evidence would suffice.

The decision to focus on the lives of Sima Vaisman, Louis Micheels and Gisella Perl was the result of three factors: the doctors had (a) written an autobiography or memoir; (b) represented a spread of gender and age, and (c) had living relatives who were willing to be interviewed. The experiences and actions of a further two Jewish doctors who survived Auschwitz, Alina Brewda and Lucie Adelsberger and one, Maximilian Samuel, a controversial figure who did not survive, were examined in less detail, primarily as I was unable to establish contact with any of their family members. Work on this book began in Auschwitz and continued at Yad Vashem in Israel; it then took me back to Warsaw and Auschwitz, to Bad Arolsen (ITS) in Germany, to the United States Holocaust Memorial Museum (USHMM) in Washington, and eventually to New York and Boston. Among the millions of archival documents in these libraries and museums many were crucial to my research. Unfortunately, I could find no living Jewish doctors who had survived Auschwitz to meet and interview. Instead I contacted and interviewed family members and friends of these survivors: I spoke to Gisele Perl's daughter Ellie and her grandson Giora; to Louis Micheels' wife Ina and their son and daughter Ron and Elizabeth; and to Sima Vaisman's nephews and nieces, Emanuel, Nadia, Diane and many friends. The respondents shared life experiences they had shared with them or had personally observed in the survivors during the pre-war years, the period in the ghettoes, transit camps and Auschwitz, and post-war years. I approached the respondents with specific questions but allowed them to talk freely about anything pertaining to the subject. They were keen to express their thoughts, feelings and observations concerning their survivor relative and receptive to further discussions after our initial meeting. I received valuable and, in some cases, completely new information.

I turned to historiography that provided me with important information about the camp, its establishment, conditions within the camp, the culture of cruelty and evil, and the health and medical system of the camp. The most valuable resources were the memoirs from which I gained an intimate knowledge of the doctors' ordeals, actions, and behaviour, enabling me to create a construct explaining survival. While memoirs are not considered to be an unquestionable source of facts, I took the approach that if I encountered the same account time after time from an array of both doctors and ordinary prisoners, it was likely to be true. For instance, if every memoir gave an almost identical description of the atrocious and inhumane conditions on the cattle trains, I was forced to believe the truth of the statements and the conditions.

As I read and reread their memoirs, patterns began to emerge that made sense of the marvel of their survival. There were patterns in the life stories the doctors told regarding their childhood and family life, religious teaching, the antisemitism they suffered, losses and successes they experienced, their experiences at medical school, in transit camps and ghettoes and their eventual life in Auschwitz. Their stories of survival are representative of most of the Jewish doctor survivors I studied. Unsurprisingly, the primary and most commanding premise for survival to emerge from the memoirs was the single-minded will to live. What mattered most to the survivors was life itself. Renowned psychiatrist and Holocaust survivor Viktor Frankl posits that finding meaning in life, a reason to live, allows endurance and survival of even the most dehumanizing and torturous conditions. On commencing treatment of a patient with depression, Frankl would ask the patient why they had not committed suicide if they were so depressed. The response would provide him with what the patient saw as their meaning in life. When I asked the Holocaust survivors I interviewed why they had survived, many responded with answers such as: 'to see my mother again,' 'to marry my childhood girlfriend,' 'to bear witness to the atrocities,' and so on. For the thirteen-year-old 'Mengele twin' Kalman Bar-On, whose story of survival is addressed in Chapter 6 the meaning in his life was to protect his mother and twin sister by ensuring they had sufficient food to eat and clothing to protect themselves from the elements. As the philosopher Friedrich Nietzsche was want to say, 'where there is a why there is a how'. Thus, the will to live was the foundation for the material, emotional and psychological pillars, the how by which survivor doctors maintained their physical health, sustained their emotional health and kept mentally active and functional. To survive the first needs that had to be met were the essentials of life: food, water, clothing and shelter. Starvation and freezing conditions killed hundreds of thousands of prisoners but with their new role in the hospitals and infirmaries the doctors acquired *status* and became *privileged* prisoners entitled to more food, better clothing and accommodation.

The second pillar for survival, identified from the memoirs and interviews with family members, was possessing important lifesaving *personal traits*. Resilience, hardiness, determination, self-esteem and perseverance were some of the traits needed to cope with the conditions and suffering. Research has found that early socialization, family culture and personal experience play a significant role in moulding these characteristics. The survivors were not suddenly endowed with these traits upon entering Auschwitz; they were a product of both nature and nurture.

The third pillar was having a defence *mechanism*. Usually this defence mechanism was work, and its role was twofold: First, a task that preoccupied the doctor or became a distraction, even if for a brief period the prisoner was given respite from fear, anxiety and physical harm. Work could also be a form a resistance that in turn could be interpreted as an expression of dignity that enhanced self-esteem. Second, the task would give the prisoner a meaning to life albeit a tenuous one. To survive Auschwitz prisoner doctors needed all of these components to coexist.

Prisoners in Auschwitz lost everything a normal person would consider 'natural' in life; they lost their identities and families and were removed from their relationships, cultural roots, and the structures and sense of security that had previously maintained them. For the prisoner in Auschwitz life began once again as a defenceless weak body in all of its' nakedness – humanity at its most vulnerable. As Shakespeare's *King* Lear observes looking at the tragic emaciated Poor Tom begging in the street:

> Why, thou wert better in thy grave than to answer with thy
> Uncovered body this extremity of the skies. – Is man no
> more than this? Consider him well. – Thou owest the
> worn no silk, the beast no hide, the sheep no wool, the cat
> no perfume. Ha! Here's three on's are sophisticated.
> Thou art the thing itself.
> Unaccommodated man is no more but such a poor, bare,
> Forked animal as thou art. (Shakespeare 1963, Act 3, Scene 4)

Under extreme adversity the human body with all of its frailties and vulnerability to harm determines our existence. The body was the prisoners' only possession and their bodies failed them. For the vast majority, sickness, starvation, beatings, the elements and exhaustion were the causes of death. In civilized circumstances most people have networks, relationships and structure to lead them through crises. In Auschwitz, inmates were isolated within the uncertainty and insecurity of life under a death sentence. Only very few were able to steer their way through that maze and find the resilience and determination to take advantage of whatever opportunities presented themselves in order to survive. Some of these few were Jewish doctors.

—

Part I: **The Road to Auschwitz**

As a religion, Judaism has long countenanced it [medicine] as a respectable and indeed nec-
essary calling, and socially the Jews have long viewed medicine as a path to professional ful-
filment and honour within the community. (Efron 2001, 2)

The road taken by Jewish doctors to Auschwitz is a cautionary tale and an example of how forces experienced throughout life shape who we are and prepare us for what we will face. It is a cautionary tale because at the beginning of the twentieth century the western European Jews were largely accepted, even had assimilated into society yet within forty-five years they were the victims of genocide. Second by following the path taken by the Jewish doctors over the period from 1900 to 1945, particularly those who survived, we become witnesses to how the past through nurture and nature determines human strengths and weaknesses. Although history is not tangible it is a beacon that should protect and prevent historical events that include genocide, the violation of human rights, terrorism and racism from being repeated. Thus, it is important to have some understanding of the life and trials and tribulations experienced by the average Jewish person and the Jewish doctor during the forty years leading up to the Final Solution.

Prior to the Holocaust, the Jewish doctors of Europe were largely assimilated in their respective societies and considered themselves citizens of the countries in which they and their families were born and lived. Memoirs, oral testimonies and biographies suggest they belonged to close-knit families and communities that valued relationships, family ties, education, religious observance and ad-herence and respect to the laws of the state. The communities were characterized by several distinctive attributes, most of which still hold true today. They were dependent on strong attachments, both on the familial and on the community level. There was close spatial interaction, as orthodox and, in particular, ultra-orthodox Jews must live within walking distance from a synagogue or *mikva* (ritual bath) and close to their extended family for the purpose of gatherings on the Sabbath, holy days and festivals. There was a strong commitment to keeping the family together – for the young and aged to live together and for children to care for their parents and other members of the extended family and to partici-pate in Jewish organizations and associations, particularly ones that extended help to those in need.

It becomes clear that early life experiences, particularly the influence of family life, the encouragement and determination to receive an education, and, in most cases, the commitment to practice their faith and the refusal to bow down to antisemitism influenced the survivors' later life attitudes and responses to challenges they were to face. Although they were considered a group on the pe-riphery of society throughout history, Jewish doctors established themselves as

https://doi.org/10.1515/9783110598216-002

a successful part of the society wherever they settled and in almost every sphere of medicine including research, pioneers in specialization, the establishment of clinics and hospitals, and health insurance. Since emancipation and despite discrimination and antisemitism, they had achieved heights of success nationally and internationally. From the turn of the century to 1936, eight Jews from Germany, Austria and Russia were recipients of the prestigious Nobel Prize for scientific and medical research.[9]

By the early 1930s, more than half of all Nobel prizes in science had been awarded to German-speaking scientists while many of the most advanced medical tools and concepts had been developed in Germany (Proctor, 1988, 293). Research contributed to innovations and medical progress that allowed such countries as Germany and Austria to be considered centres of medical and scientific excellence. According to Saul Friedländer (1997, 225),

> on April 1, 1933, some 8000 to 9000 Jewish physicians were practicing in Germany. By the end of 1934, approximately 2,200 had either migrated or abandoned their profession, but despite their steady decline during 1935, at the beginning of 1936, 5000 Jewish physicians (among them 2,800 in the Public Health Service) were still working in the Reich.

By early 1939 this number had been reduced to 285 (Kater 1989, 201). The tragic loss of doctors by emigration, suicide, murder and incarceration symbolized the death of German Jewry in that the Jewish doctor represented everything the Jews aspired to and had achieved in Germany. They were successful in the professions (law, medicine, finance), in business (trade, manufacturing, small business), in scholarship (university, research and teaching) and politics. They had assimilated into the society and at the same time continued to practice their religion. Germany from the middle of the nineteenth century had become the centre of medical research and scholarship attracting researchers, academics and medical students worldwide. After the enlightenment[10] Germany encouraged the

---

9 Nobel Prize recipients: 1908 Paul Ehrlich, Germany, Erie Metchnikoff, Russia, 1914 Robert Barany Austria, 1922 Otto Meyerhof, Germany, 1930 Karl Landsteiner, Austria, 1931 Otto Warburg, Germany, 1936 Otto Loewi, Austria. Ernst Chain, a recipient in 1945, had fled to Britain in 1933 believing it was not safe for a Jew in Hitler's Germany (ed. Berger 1995, 234).

10 The Enlightenment began as a secularizing intellectual movement among thinkers and writers in the seventeenth century. The movement concentrated on a change in attitude and values less tied to tradition with an emphasis on a more liberal open-minded approach in society. Although this movement developed political overtones with a focus on turning royal absolutism into a form of democratic republicanism it first entered the world stage with minor interest or appeal from the masses. In fact antisemitism, discrimination and violence towards the Jews continued. By contrast there was a growing view by the Radical Enlightenment that the narrow

development of a Jewish health care system with hospitals, clinics and medical training. The Jewish physician and medical services were highly regarded and attracted both Jewish and non-Jewish patients. As John Efron (2001, 3) states, 'few occupations are as immediately linked to a group as medicine is to the Jews ... and ... as a people, the Jews have enjoyed an intimate and deeply symbiotic relationship with medicine.' However, there is no doubt that the irrefutable success of the Jewish doctor, particularly from the turn of the century, contributed to the increasing level of resentment, discontentment and, finally, outright antisemitism felt by Aryan doctors.

At the turn of the nineteenth century, Jews constituted approximately two per cent of Germany's doctors, however, by the beginning of the twentieth century, Jews, who represented just over one per cent of the German population made up sixteen per cent of Germany's doctors (Efron 2001, 234). Approximately one third of medical doctors in Berlin were Jewish. According to Efron (2001, 234), medicine had become so fundamental 'to the social structure and thus self-perception of German Jewry that nearly one half of all Jews attending universities in 1900 studied medicine.' Jewish women made up a very high proportion of the women attending European medical schools especially in Germany (Freidenreich 1996, 80). The universities of Germany not only experienced an influx of German Jews into the faculties of medicine. Due to the manifest antisemitic quota systems, which limited the number of Jews who could study medicine in countries such as Poland and Russia, there was a continuous stream of foreign students into German universities. The extent of this migration of foreign students is demonstrated by the figures for the University of Königsberg, at which by 1911 foreign Jews studying medicine outnumbered German Jews. While foreign Jews had constituted a mere seven per cent of all Jewish university students that figure skyrocketed to fifty-six per cent by 1911–1912 (Efron 2001, 235). In Vienna approximately fifty per cent of the city's doctors and sixty-three per cent of dentists were Jewish. Similarly, in Poland some 3,500 Jewish doctors accounted for almost twenty per cent of the country's approximately 20,000 physicians (ed. Falstein 1963, 46).

The hostility and alienation towards the Jewish doctors that had begun fermenting since the turn of the century increased at the end of the Great War. Germany's defeat had destroyed the country politically, socially and economically, and the new government, the Weimar Republic, was weak and unable to provide stability and security. Under the Republic the seeds of xenophobia,

---

occupation structure imposed on the Jews was imposing stifling and intolerant restrictions and disabilities on the Jews. Starting with the French Revolution there arose the phenomenon of the revolutionary Jew adopting the principles of this radical Enlightenment.

racism and antisemitism took root and flourished. Antagonism towards the Jews grew in direct relationship to their involvement, perceived influence and integration into German politics, finance, culture and business. The most successful became the most vulnerable and Jewish doctors were confronted 'with an antisemitic campaign of remarkable vehemence' (Efron 2001, 5). In a country with a destroyed economy and chronic unemployment, the combination of thousands of German physicians returning home from the War and the arrival of hundreds of immigrant Jewish doctors fleeing from pogroms in Tsarist Russia led to fierce competition for work within the medical profession. When over time it became obvious that the Jewish doctor were more successful at finding work than German doctors, they begun to be perceived as a serious threat to the continuing livelihood of the German doctors, especially medical graduates seeking work. The success of the Jewish doctor by way of competency and providing better health services attributed to the rise in unemployment of non-Jewish doctors and dentists. Despite the bitterness and ill-feeling there was little that could be done to curb Jewish domination. It was not until Hitler came to power in 1933 that the German doctor saw some hope that their professional and financial status would improve and measures would be taken to rid them of Jewish competition.

Antisemitism existed in Germany before the Nazis came to power yet it was relatively mild compared to that suffered by Jews in neighbouring countries such as Poland, Hungary, France, and Russia. Nevertheless, the pervading atmosphere of blatant discrimination created by the imminent coming to power of an antisemitic regime gave local councils and municipalities, universities and other institutions license to begin discriminatory actions against Jews. At the same time the popular press and medical journals openly condemned the continuing influence and monopoly of Jews in the country's medical system. Hitler's accession to power and the National Socialist takeover in 1933 was a watershed and marked the end of the German government's adherence to legal norms which had offered Jews some measure of protection in the preceding years' (Wildt 2000, 183). Once the Law for the Reconstruction of the Civil Services[11] was introduced in 1933, even

---

[11] The Law for the Restoration of the Professional Civil Service (Gesetz zur Wiederherstellung des Berufsbeamtentums, shortened to Berufsbeamtengesetz), also known as Civil Service Law, Civil Service Restoration Act, and Law to Re-establish the Civil Service, was presented on 7 April 1933, immediately after Hitler became Chancellor. The law gave the government the power to dismiss tenured civil servants including opponents of the Nazi regime, undesirables and civil servants who were not of "Aryan descent". This meant Jews and political opponents would be forced to retire or would be dismissed. This included lawyers, teachers, academics, judges and all public servants.

tenured civil servants of non-Aryan descent could be legally dismissed. Local government officials of Berlin and Munich, Julius Lippert, State Commissioner of Berlin, and Karl Fiehler, Mayor of Munich, respectively, of their own accord broke legitimate contracts when they dismissed all Jewish public health and welfare physicians (Kater 1989, 185). In Bavaria the contracts of Jewish doctors working for the public-school system were dismissed and in Munich Jewish doctors could only treat Jewish patients. In Hamburg after 1933:

> [the city's] community welfare administration had operated according to the tenor and spirit of National Socialism from the outset. It not only accepted the creation of a completely new welfare group, the Jews, but also contributed of its own accord and finally actively practiced discrimination and segregation. (Lohalm 2000, 45)

Kurt Klare, co-founder of the Nazi Physicians' League, wrote to a colleague Dr Scheidegg, 'that Jews and philosemites ought to take note of the fact that Germans are masters of their own house once more and will control their own destiny' (Kater 1989, 183). Another founder of the League, Dr Conti, warned that because no professional group in Germany had been harmed more by Jewry than the medical one, nobody ought to be surprised when Hitler effectively orchestrated the gradual disenfranchisement of the Jewish doctor in German medicine. He appointed Dr Gerhard Wagner, The Führer's Commissioner for National Health, to oversee the reorganization and restructure of the German medical system, and it was Wagner aided by Carl Haedenkamp and Alfons Stauder who initiated the process for dismissing Jewish functionaries from the national medical associations as well as regional and local groups (Kater 1989, 183). From May 17, 1934 Jewish doctors were no longer allowed to be a member of and practice within Germany's state-supported health insurance program. This was, in fact, a sequel to the Law for the Reconstruction of the Civil Services of April 7, 1933 that effectively removed all Jewish physicians (Amtsärzte) from the civil service. During 1934 and 1935 pharmacists and dentists were targeted and had to show proof of Aryan descent. Legislation began to have a far-reaching and permanent impact on the Jewish physician when the Reich Physicians' Ordinance of December 13, 1935 was introduced. Gentiles were forbidden to be treated by Jewish doctors or to attend a Jewish hospital. Jewish doctors were forbidden to call themselves 'physicians' and only allowed to use the more degrading term, 'sick treaters' (Efron 2001, 264).

This progressive erosion of the recognition Jewish doctors in the Reich reached its conclusion with the legislation of the Fourth Ordinance of the Citizen Law, enacted on July 25, 1938, which revoked the medical licenses of Jewish physicians thus preventing them from practicing medicine in Germany. Despite the early rush in 1933 to victimize and discriminate against Jewish doctors, at 'the end of September (1938), then, Jewish doctors, as the world had admired them for decades, to all intents and purposes vanished from the German medical scene' (Kater 1989, 200). The process evolved over a five-year period through a combination of propaganda, intimidation and official laws. Jewish doctors were accused of sexual assault by German women patients, their surgeries and clinic leases were revoked or not renewed, those holding academic positions, some eminent international medical scientists were dismissed, they were accused of monopolizing the medical profession and causing financial hardship to German doctors and their families. Subsequently the doctors became victims of pogroms during which, 'in accordance with the "Aryan" medical counterculture that wished to see Jews dead, were, if anything, treated more brutally than non-doctors because they alone could help preserve Jewish life'(Kater 1989, 201).

Joseph Tenenbaum argues that in the post-Great-War period Poland was borne on a wave of pogroms where Jew-baiting, Jew-beating, beard-cutting and economic discrimination was endemic (Tenenbaum 1963, 144). According to Edmund Goldenberg (1995), a survivor of Auschwitz, born in Terezin, Czechoslovakia, but educated in Poland, antisemitism was unrestrained and widespread throughout Poland, nowhere more so than in the schools and universities. Goldenberg recalled that at Kacimierz University, there was a quota system with a limit of ten per cent Jews. The student body and teaching staff were extremely antisemitic. Jewish students were not allowed to sit or communicate with non-Jews and various humiliations were introduced by actively antisemitic professors. One such was:

> the 'ghetto bench,' an arrangement whereby Jews were allowed to sit only in a special area on the left side of the lecture hall. Another was the placing of yellow tags on those benches, bearing the resurrected medieval slogan, 'Here sits a Jew'. (Roland 1992, 9)

According to Janina Zaborowska, a non-Jewish medical student, there was physical intimidation at Warsaw University, including the beating of Jews with rubber hoses in the dissecting room (Roland 1992, 9). Goldenberg (1995) maintains that Jewish students were even required to find their own corpses to carry out dissections. He suggests that prior to the invasion the Polish government and the institutions were watching the events in Germany under Hitler and trying to implement similar policies that discriminated against the Jewish doctors. This is important in regards to the working relationship of medical staff in Auschwitz because Jewish doctors not only needed to fear the Nazi SS in the camp, they were forced to contend with bullying, humiliation and sometimes beatings by non-Jewish prisoners, particularly Polish doctors. Jewish doctors in all Nazi-occupied countries suffered a similar fate. Professor Josef Charvát, a Czechoslovakian endocrinologist and specialist in general internal diseases, who was a prisoner doctor in Dachau, writes of the poor sanitary conditions and the fate of medicine in Czechoslovakia under German occupancy:

> All the universities (which in our country also educated medical doctors) were closed down by force on the 17th November 1939, and for fully six years we were without any possibility of educating and training medical practitioners. Many Czech doctors were arrested, sent to concentration camps or executed; all Jewish doctors were deported and most of them done away with (*Medical Science Abused: German Medical Science as Practiced in Concentration Camps and in the so-called Protectorate* 1946).

The ghettos introduced the Jewish doctors to conditions that were beyond their comprehension. Epidemics were rampant, typhoid and malaria for example were foreign to many doctors, particularly young graduates, medicine and equipment was almost non-existent, and many doctors were not qualified in the fields of medicine most needed. Starvation was at the core of almost every illness. The quantity and quality of food and water was so poor as to cause massive weight loss and emaciation, which led to the breakdown of the immune system, which in turn led to epidemics and chronic diarrhoea. The population of the ghetto of Warsaw was approximately five hundred thousand Jews, Lodz ghetto alone housing a population of approximately three hundred and twenty thousand. Essentially, the plan was to empty the countryside of Jews and drive them into the city precincts and the walled ghettos. This led to overcrowding, massive unemployment, disease and epidemics. Some of the true perspective of the conditions that prevailed is demonstrated by these statistics:

> [O]ne third of the population of the entire city of Warsaw...was crammed into the ghetto, which took up no more than three to four percent of the built area of the city. People were crowded seven to a room. The ghetto was in the poorest vicinity of Warsaw; the problems exacerbated by the run-down environment, cramped streets and deficient drainage. (Nadav 2009, 70)

The official food allocation in the Warsaw ghetto gives an even more indication of the inadequacy: Polish prisoners received 634 calories per day and 2310 for the Germans (Noakes & Prindham 1988, 1067). Thus to survive was very difficult. The following are descriptions of life in the ghettos and camps that provide an insight into the conditions in which the Jewish doctor and carer were required to work. Stanislav Rozycki, a visitor to the Warsaw ghetto provides evidence of these conditions:

> The majority are nightmare figures, ghosts of former human beings, miserable destitutes, pathetic remnants of former humanity. One is most affected by the characteristic change which one sees in their faces: as a result of misery, poor nourishment, lack of vitamins,

fresh air and exercise, the numerous cares, worries, anticipated misfortunes, suffering and sickness, their faces have taken on a skeletal appearance...On the streets children are crying in vain, children who are dying of hunger. They howl, beg, sing, moan, shiver with cold, without underwear, without clothing, without shoes, in rags, sacks, flannel which are bound in strips round emancipated skeletons, children swollen with hunger, disfigured, half conscious, already completely grown up at the age of five, gloomy and weary of life...The fatal over-population is particularly apparent in the streets: people literally rub against each other, it is impossible to pass unhindered through the streets. (Noakes & Prindham 1988, 1067)

Alfred Rosenberg[12]visiting the Lublin and Warsaw ghettos wrote to the Reich press:

[T]his race en masse, which is decaying, decomposing and rotten to the core will banish any sentimental humanitarianism. In the Warsaw ghetto there are at present fifty typhus cases a month and one cannot ascertain how many are not reported. Seven hundred Jewish doctors have been put in the ghetto who live there and have to concentrate on fighting typhus...The Warsaw ghetto contains five hundred thousand Jews of whom five to six thousand die each month. In reply to my question as to whether it was reckoned that in ten years-time the Jews would be finished through having died off, Dr. Frank said he did not want to wait that long. (Noakes & Prindham 1988, 1069)

Both the doctor and the hospital were revered in the ghetto, the former as a healer and protector and the latter as the nerve centre of the ghetto. Unlike the concentration camps where the hospitals were considered transit houses to the gas chambers, the ghetto hospital was the *Hekdesh*, a refuge for the sick, the destitute and the old. The hospital was also a safe haven for the underground:

[T]he hospital not only presented an acceptable facade but concealed behind the facade a multitude of forbidden and illegal underground activities...If we assume that the word 'resistance' includes all activities aimed at preserving the values which the enemy intends to destroy, then it is no exaggeration to say that the hospital was a bastion of resistance in the ghetto...this is how the *Hekdesh* became a fortress...[13]

As time passed the conditions within the ghettos became worse, which led to increased starvation and epidemics and even higher death rates. Ludwik Hirszfeld, a serologist, who served on the Health Council of the Warsaw ghetto, was convinced that the sanitary conditions in the ghetto were an intentional prelude to the murderous intentions of the Nazis: 'When one concentrates

---

12 Alfred Rosenberg was an influential Nazi racial philosopher. His writing included the 1930 book "The Myth of the Twentieth Century" which declared the existence of two opposing races: the Aryan race, creator of all values and culture and the Jewish race, the agent of cultural corruption – a viewpoint taken literally by Hitler and National Socialist ideology.

13 Wajnryb. Ibid. p. 39.

400,000 wretches in one district, takes everything away from them, and gives them nothing, then one creates typhus' (Weindling 2000, 280). It is within this context that Jewish doctors with an overwhelming number of sick and undernourished patients and virtually no resources were required to work. Dvorjetski, a survivor of the Vilna ghetto, saw the Jewish physicians as guardians of life, thwarting Nazi intentions of exterminating ghetto inhabitants by means of epidemics (Dvorjetski 1952, 280). In ghettos such as Warsaw medical research was conducted and medical education was provided in the form of the continuation of university studies. Apart from their obvious value, these clandestine activities were a form of spiritual resistance. Lack of food was the fundamental problem of the ghetto, which could not be solved because of rationing and Nazi policy of limiting food supplies into the ghetto. The governor of the Generalgouvernement, Hans Frank, predicted unequivocally that the Nazis had condemned 1,200,000 Jews to death by starvation (Roland 1992, 101). In the face of malnutrition and starvation as the primary condition they could not alleviate, the medical community of the Warsaw ghetto saw the opportunity to carry out research on the disease. As Milejkowski, one of the originators of the hunger disease project explains:

> Hunger was the most important factor of everyday life within the wall of Warsaw ghetto. Its symptoms consisted of crowds of beggars and corpses often lying in the streets covered with newspapers. Mortality data on hunger and its two companions, tuberculosis and typhus, were collected from orphanages and refugee centres and from specific hospital material. (Winick 1997, 4)

The results of this study, which are still used as source of reference today, were smuggled out of the ghetto and have been widely published. Further experiments of great value were carried out on other diseases, such as typhus. Dvorjetski (1952) quotes Israel Mileijkovsky as addressing his fellow doctors in 1942 whilst in the Warsaw ghetto as follows:

> To you, Jewish doctors, some modest words of acknowledgement. What should I tell you, dear friend and partner to suffering? Your fate is the fate of all; slavery, famine, deportations – those all are the death figures in our Ghetto – which had not passed you over. And you, by your work, gave the only answer to the murderers. Here goes the answer: NON OMNIS MORIAR! (not all of me will die!).

Antisemitism had always been a fundamental part of Jewish life. The beginning of the twentieth century introduced a new and completely different dimension to the meaning of antisemitism which over a relative short period became an attempt to commit genocide. From the shelter of a culture that valued family, education, faith in God, community and peace, the Jews of Europe were gradually immersed into a sewer of inhumanity and evil they could never have anticipated or imagined. A group who were one of the first to feel the wrath of a new type of antisemitism and then the fury of Nazism were the Jewish doctors in Germany. They were hounded from their profession by their non-Jewish colleagues and then prevented from practicing medicine under Hitler's racial laws. They were among the first Jews to be sent to concentration and labour camps and among the first to be selected for execution on the basis they were considered intellectuals, a threat to National Socialism. Those doctors who failed or refused to leave Germany or other countries soon to be occupied by Nazi when given the opportunity were sent to ghettoes and then concentration and death camps. Only a very small number of Jewish doctors survived the Holocaust.

When they arrived at the ghettoes and camps many doctors that survived did not suddenly find the personal traits of resilience, hardiness, self-esteem, determination or the indestructible will to live. Their past shaped their actions and reactions – socialization, experiences, family influences, education, failures and successes and natural traits.

Part II: Parallel Lives: Drs Sima Vaisman, Gisella Perl and Louis Micheels

Rejected by mankind, the condemned do not go so far as to reject it in turn. Their faith in history remain unshaken, and one may well wonder why. They do not despair. The proof: they persist in surviving – not only to survive, but to testify. The victims elect to become witnesses. (Des Pres 1976, 28)

Who were these Jewish doctors who survived such extreme adversity, and what gave them the capacity to do so? Did they have extraordinary energy and skills? Did they possess exceptional personal traits that allowed them to overcome their situation and rise above the emotional and psychological trauma? Did the forces that shaped them as children prepare them for what would confront them in adulthood? Shaping forces are an important part of survival that includes both nature and nurture. And of course in a place such as Auschwitz when life and death was so unpredictable luck and the lawless power of accident played a significant role ruling over the fate of all prisoners.

The character of the books is as diverse as the history of the authors. There is constant anguish and foreboding by Micheels *117646 A Holocaust Memoir: A Psychoanalyst moving account of his experience in the Nazi death camp*; there is Perl's story of betrayal by Mengele and abuse by fellow prisoners and her ability to rise above these traumatic events as she told in *I was a prisoner in Auschwitz*; there is Cohen's complex and guilt ridden memoir in the *Abyss: a Confession and Vaisman's symbolic story which conveys both wretched misery and hardened anger*. Nyiszli's *Auschwitz: A Doctor's Eyewitness Account* delivers an impersonal almost disconnected account of life in the camp where as a doctor business continued as usual. Every memoir tells a story but while in truth each one of the survivors was a doctor in reality every doctor was human. As doctors they were directed by ethics, morality and nurture. As people they were driven by reality and nature; the will to live and the want to survive. The doctors faced dilemmas; ethical, moral and religious when treating and protecting patients and following SS orders nevertheless confronted choiceless choices when their own lives were threatened. As normal people under enormous adversity they were influenced by the human condition. Survival of extreme adversity over an extended period as experienced by POWs, hostages, prisoners of death camps and so on does not just happen. To repeat what I have said the Jewish doctors who survived Auschwitz lived an average of two years before liberation. Under such utter barbarity and pitilessness how did their urge to live win over the wish to die? The words of the survivors will help to put together the jigsaw of a complex array of factors that assisted them to escape and win.

https://doi.org/10.1515/9783110598216-003

1 Dr Sima Vaisman

It was in Brezinka that I fell into the heart of hell.
Sima Vaisman (2005, 52)

Sima Vaisman (Wasserman) was born in 1902 in Kishinev, Bessarabia, Moldavia, where she lived with her parents, Fraiche and Mania Wasserman (née Weinberg) and her younger sister, Rachel. Jews had been living in Bessarabia since the 14th century. After Sephardic merchants began trading in the 15th century, commerce between Polish-Jewish merchants increased steadily. During the 19th century the Jewish population of Bessarabia grew from approximately 20,000 to over 200,000, a development encouraged by Tzar Nicholas I. The Tsar granted tax incentives for Jews to migrate and work in the rural areas of the Bessarabia region, where Tsarist authorities created 17 Jewish agricultural colonies. At the beginning of the 20th century, Jewish life in the governorate of Bessarabia[14] was flourishing with a population of over 228,000 Jews (Weiner 1999). Many were active and successful in commerce, particularly in liquor distilling and agriculture. Despite the Jewish community being allowed to lead an active religious and cultural life, antisemitism existed and pogroms were increasingly common. Bessarabian Jews were subject to vicious attacks in 1870, between 1903 and 1905, and again in 1905 to 1906. In one of the two most infamous pogroms that took place between 1903 and 1905, arguably the first state-sponsored pogrom of the 20th century, forty-seven Jews in Kishinev were killed and hundreds injured.[15]

The early life of Sima was a happy one. Like most young girls she and her sister enjoyed a normal childhood, with many friends and acquaintances engaging in regular social activities. Her father was a successful scrap metal merchant so the family was reasonably prosperous. Her mother Mania was a devoted and loving wife and mother. The girls attended school, and the family was surrounded by many relatives and friends, most of whom were Jewish. When Sima was twelve, her father died from tetanus. The family suffered financially and went to live with the Halfins, the family of Mania's sister Sarah. Sarah's husband Shmaya was a well-to-do merchant,

---

14 Bessarabia is the geographic region in Eastern Europe bounded by the Dniester River and the Prut River on the east. Since the beginning of the nineteenth century Bessarabia has been occupied, either by Russia, Romania or Moldova. After WWII Moldova was claimed by the Soviet Union and it was not until 1990 that free democratic elections were held. Moldavian SSR became SSR Moldova and later the Republic of Moldova. During WWII it was occupied by the Soviet Union and Romania. Romania was an ally of the Germans. Romania co-operated with the Nazis in their drive to rid Europe of Jews actively taking part in the Final Solution.
15 The second major pogrom took place during the civil war (1918–1921) between the Bolsheviks and their opponents in which some 35,000 Jews were killed and over 100,000 Jews were left homeless.

https://doi.org/10.1515/9783110598216-004

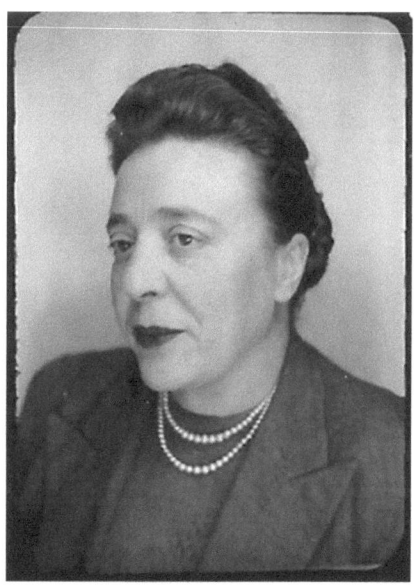

Fig. 1: Dr. Sima Vaisman before the Holocaust. (from the private collection of Sima Vaisman's extended family and friends).

and they lived with their children Bella, Bouma (Abraham) and Leon in a spacious house in Kishinev. Sima and Rachel attended school with their cousins and occasionally enjoyed summer vacations in Carlsbad, Bohemia. Sima was a gifted and highly motivated scholar. Despite the *numerus clausus*,[16] introduced to limit the number of Jews admitted to study medicine, she gained entry to the medical school in Bucharest. Sima stayed with another of Mania's sisters, Fanny, and her husband Moisey Galperin, for the duration of her studies. She graduated with honours, specializing in gynaecology, and began working in a hospital in Bucharest. The above photograph, Fig. 1., is of Sima as a doctor before the the war in her late 30s according to her relatives. To have qualified as doctor despite these social and political challenges attests to Sima's extraordinary resilience, confidence and determination, characteristics that would prove invaluable in her later life.

In the late 1920s, Sima was introduced to Paul Vaisman, an electrical engineer, originally from Kishinev who was living in Paris, during one of his visits home. They were married in the early 1930s and moved to Paris. Since her medical degree from Bucharest was not recognized in France, and to re-qualify as a medical doctor was expensive, Sima retrained as a dentist. She and her husband were happy in Paris and life was good. However, toward the end of the 1930s, life

---

16 This restricted number of Jews to enrol and attend university. This was common policy throughout most European countries before they became occupied Nazi territory.

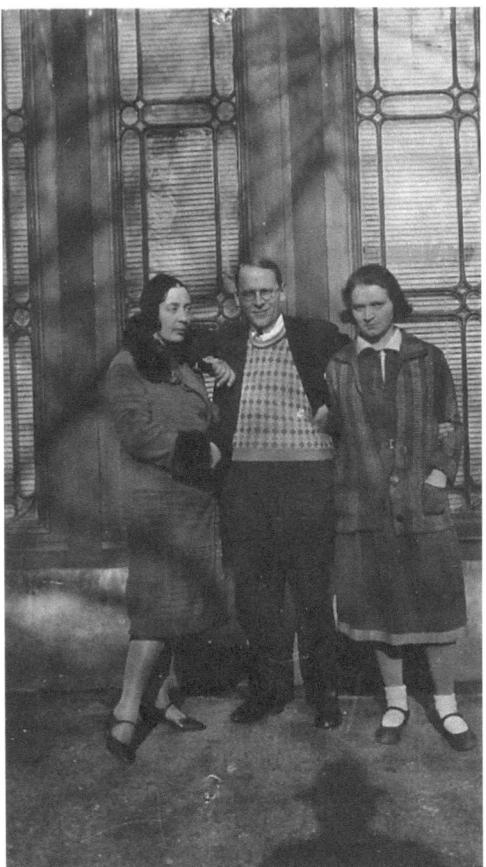

Fig. 2: Sima with husband Paul and sister Rachel.(from the private collection of Sima Vaisman's extended family and friends).

would change irrevocably. In 1937 Paul was diagnosed with lymphoma and died that year. With the beginning of World War II and the occupation of France, there was a dramatic rise in antisemitism. Life in Paris became ever more difficult for Jews. Sima fled to the south of France hoping to escape the discrimination, violence and deportations, but was arrested by the French militia in Saône-et-Loire on 23 December 1943 and handed over to the Gestapo in Lyon. From Lyon, she was transferred to Drancy internment camp outside Paris, from where some 65,000 Jews would eventually be deported to the extermination and labour camps in the east. Sima Vaisman was 42 years old when she was deported on 20 January 1944, along with 1,155 fellow Jews. They were loaded onto cattle cars where they spent three days and two nights slowly rolling towards their destination, Auschwitz.

> Sixty people per car, men, women and children crammed together; on the ground a few
> dirty straw mattresses, a tin chamber pot, a bucket of water ... The doors to the car are
> sealed; we settle ourselves in the dark as best we can and the journey to the unknown
> begins ... Auschwitz, land of death ... The 'die of fate' is cast, we must submit to it and hold
> strong, hold strong above all. (Vaisman 2005, 28)

For Vaisman the life she had known before National Socialism poisoned Europe
vanished; instead she found herself in a foreign and frightening situation. Even
before arriving in Auschwitz, she appears to have known that in order to survive she
would need to be strong now and at all times, whatever may happen. This is the first
sign of Sima's resilience and determination to survive. On arrival at the camp on 22
January, the SS ordered doctors and single women without families to step forward.
Vaisman joined the fifty-five young women (nos. 74783-74797 – 74835-74874) and
two hundred and thirty-six men (nos. 172611-172846) selected to go to the right while
the remaining 864 men, women and children were loaded onto trucks (Czech 1990,
575). She was later to learn that they had been sent to the gas chambers. This was
a 'normal' day in Auschwitz. Ironically, being alone when she arrived in Auschwitz
and having no relatives or friends whose immediate fate she was concerned about
was an advantage. Although she would obviously have feared for the fate of her
mother, sister and extended family, she did not have to witness them at the gates of
Auschwitz, being led to the gas or thrown into the fire pits.

Following selection, Vaisman (2005, 30) and her fellow prisoners were subjected to the next process of degradation and humiliation. They were tattooed,
shorn of all body hair, and showered.

> [A]fter the shower (no towel), we go into a large cold room, ice-cold, with a cement floor,
> where other girls hand out to us those poor rags that will henceforth have to serve us as
> our clothes, rags to wrap our feet in, old worn out shoes that are too small or too big. They
> paint red crosses on these miserable clothes, symbol of this heavy cross we will have to bear.
> (Vaisman 2005, 28)[17]

The SS provided the women clothes that were nothing more than rags. They were
humiliated and unrecognizable becoming nothing more than a number. This
process was part of SS policy to dehumanize the prisoners and to break them

---

17 The red cross was designed and first painted on the back of prisoners' clothing by 'Zippi'
Spitzer, a Slovakian Jewess among the first to be deported to Auschwitz's Stammlager. According
to Konrad Kwiet (2009, 16), 'Zippi' mixed the paint from vermilion, oil, turpentine and siccatives
(drying agents) and painted a two-centimetre wide cross over backs of her fellow inmates, 'from
the top to bottom; from the neck to the legs.' Kwiet contends that while tattoos have been the
subject of investigation the use of other insignia such as red stripes has not been given symbolic
meaning or little attention at all.

emotionally and psychologically to such an extent that they could not resist carrying out the orders of the SS and the Kapos. For the next three weeks Vaisman lived in filth with a shameful lack of privacy and worked in a labour squad:

> [W]e have to do excavation work, or walk two and half miles in both directions six or seven times a day, on foot, each time carrying a stone. We are accompanied by the SS followed by police dogs [*who*] hurl themselves at those of us who can no longer walk and tear them to pieces. (Vaisman 2005, 33)

This experience exposed her to the hardship and brutality prisoners in the camp endured on a daily basis. It prepared her for the next stage of camp life. After three weeks Vaisman was assigned to the *Revier* (sickbay), where typhus was rampant. The mortality rate of both prisoners and prisoner doctors was high and additional medical personnel were required. Aside from the total lack of equipment and scarcity of medications, Vaisman describes the conditions as follows:

> [N]o water, no plumbing. Light penetrates through little skylights in the ceiling. Inside, against each wall length-wise, beds ... placed end to end. Perpendicular to them, groups of two beds separated by a little space. Black dirty cots in three tiers. A repugnant straw mattress full of pus and blood with one or two blankets, and on each mattress at least two sick people, sometimes even three or four ... a smell of corpses, of excrement ... And the sick, skeletal beings, almost all covered with scabies, boils, devoured by lice, all completely naked, shivering from cold under their disgusting covers. (Vaisman 2005, 36)

The suffering was unbearable. Many years after the war, she told her niece that she had contemplated suicide during the early period. Obviously, what she witnessed scarred her emotionally and mentally. Vaisman said the Revier accommodated 3000 or 4000 sick (from a total of approximately 13,000 prisoners); roughly 300 deaths occurred per day, mainly from typhus. She worked mainly in Block 18 with patients suffering from typhoid, dysentery, malaria, hunger, oedema or thrombophlebitis.[18] Death was everywhere and occurred most commonly in the mornings. Prisoners often spent the night in misery, lying next to a corpse.

> Sometimes [it was] their mother or their sister, and thrown outside the block naked of course, into the mud or the snow according to the season ... There the piles rapidly grow. Surreal vision of these little mountains of dead bodies, covered with one single cover. Legs, arms, faces of suffering jut out on every side. (Vaisman 2005, 37)

The scenes and conditions witnessed by the Jewish doctors were soul-destroying, but not once in her memoirs is there any hint of self-pity. Despite despair and anger Vaisman accepted reality:

---

18 Related to vein inflammation potentially causing blood clotting.

[W]hat they do give us is so minimal that we consider it almost non-existent. Whether it's for the service of infections, of oedemas, or of dysentery, everyday they send us the same thing … ten aspirin tablets, ten charcoal tablets, ten tablets of urotropine, ten tablets of Tamalbrul, occasionally a syringe of cardiazol, of caffeine, or of Prontosil; a little cellulose cotton and paper strips once a week, with which to make temporary bandages. (Vaisman 2005, 38)

The haunting faces of suffering and voices begging for help gave her no respite, and she confesses that for the most part, all that could be offered were words of comfort. She recalls the struggle against lice that had spread throughout the camp and the program of delousing, 'we make our visits with scarves on our heads. When we lean over the sick women, lice fall onto our heads from the upper bunks. And the delousing was still one of the atrocious things in the camp. It was done block by block' (Vaisman 2005, 38). All prisoners including the dying, even if carried by stretcher were sent to the 'sauna' or bathhouse. Those who could still stand walked:

naked, shirtless, feet wrapped in worn-out slippers, covered with a meagre blanket, often two under one blanket that covered only their chest. Their long fleshless thighs don't touch each other, and leave enormous triangles between them. Their long legs (two thin sticks covered with a parchment skin) give way to enormous knees. They drag themselves lamentably in the snow (at times it was as cold as -15 degrees Fahrenheit) or in the mud, fall on the way, get back up under blows from batons, and drag themselves again. Faces dried up, triangular, ageless, in which only the eyes could be seen, were twisted in suffering. They shaved the ones who had head lice (and almost all of them did), showered them. Sitting on the cement floor, they waited for hours, often all night, for the blankets to be disinfected (passed under the sterilizer) and the block gassed '… on the way back, they brought the dead on stretchers. The death rate after this de-lousing was enormous, the disinfection was insufficient, and the lice continued to devour our sick'. (Vaisman 2005, 40)

Vaisman's descriptions are concise and she presents scenes of chaos and unreality. She does not reveal her role however, it must be assumed that as a Jewish doctor working in Birkenau, she was involved in the *selection* process. It seems inconceivable that *selections* occurred in some hospitals and not in others, or that some Jewish doctors were exempt from taking part in *selections*. It is left to the reader to decide if words not said have meaning. According to Nazi policy it was compulsory that every SS doctor took part in selections particularly at the time of the arrival of the trains. It becomes obvious that she along with her fellow colleagues including nurses are pro-active in protecting patients:

The personnel of the block (the medical staff was not subject to these selections) started to take out all their things, to help dress at least a few. But none of us had much to put on. Repeated searches had deprived us of a pullover, or a skirt we might have contrived to 'organize' … we quickly distribute our coats, our blouses, and our aprons. All the sick throw themselves on us, literally tear our clothes from us, beg us to give them a few rags … the few patients who had transformed themselves in this way into 'nurses' pretend to wash, to massage the sick, and to hide, as much as they can, their anxious faces from the searching eyes of our executioners ... and the commission is already there ... A silence of death ... No one dares breathe. Everyone gets out of the beds and goes to one side of the block. All the beds, all the spaces between each gap where a poor body may have hidden itself, are verified by the SS, baton in hand. Blows rain down on those they find, their numbers are recorded, their death warrant is signed ... this happens also to all the women who, having no more strength left, despite all their will, cannot get out of bed. (Vaisman 2005, 43)

Vaisman's nephew Emanuel Marom (2011) recalls that Vaisman told his daughter Edith that during a *selection* by *Hauptsturmführer* Dr Josef Mengele[19] one woman was seven months pregnant. The women were required to walk naked in front of Mengele. Vaisman organized the most beautiful woman in the group to walk in front of the pregnant woman so as to distract Mengele (who had a reputation for liking beautiful women). It worked. He didn't notice the pregnant woman who was thus saved from *selection (*Marom 2011*)*. On another occasion Vaisman saved the life of a pregnant Jewish woman whose baby had died whilst still in utero. The baby's arm and leg were protruding from her vagina. She helped the woman to properly abort the baby and avoid selection *(*Marom 2011*)*. Vaisman received privileges relative to other prisoners, such as extra clothing and food, and may have even had separate accommodation. However, she makes no mention of receiving the kinds of comfort and benefits afforded some of the Jewish doctors who worked in Block 10 such as Brewda, Samuel and Hautval, or doctors Fleck and Micheels at the Institute of Hygiene, or Nyiszli who worked for Mengele.

In April 1944 lice and typhus in Birkenau had all but been eradicated, and the Nazis commenced work on the camp to improve conditions in anticipation of Allied occupation. Vaisman (2005, 49) explains how Birkenau changed from a place of darkness and despair to one that was cleaned, sanitized and even 'beautified': 'Feverish work on plumbing begins in May. They install toilets, washrooms. The blocks are cleaned, bleached, cement floors are made where they had been only earth' (Vaisman 2005, 49). On 16 May, Vaisman was transferred to sector BIIg a camp within Birkenau consisting of forty blocks and a sauna. The camp also housed 'Kanada', the two blocks used as the collection centre of all possessions, including clothing, shoes, suitcases and personal items of those prisoners arriving at the camp. Vaisman's block had a revier, in which she had one room for what could be called consultations and another as a sick room. However, her duties

---

19 Mengele became known as Auschwitz's *Angel of Death*. He worked in the camp from May 1943 until January 1945 where he condemned hundreds of thousands of Jews to death and carried out indescribable experiments on twins, dwarfs and the disabled, mainly children. He escaped prosecution and died in Sao Paulo, Brazil, in 1978.

were not only as a doctor. It is obvious from her memoirs that she was required to carry out normal labour duties and was subject to 'Sport'.[20] Being only a matter of hundreds of meters from the crematorium and gas chambers, Sima 'fell into the very heart of hell' (Vaisman 2005, 52). From there, she was exposed to the full extent of evil. She witnessed the arrival of trains, day and night without pause.

> A few young men and women, in good health, are set apart and led to the bathhouse. They are the 'fortunate' ones, the ones chosen for a slave's 'existence' with all the wretchedness, hunger, humiliation, and slow death in shameful overcrowding ... the others are led to the gas chambers, the ovens ... and, in front of our block, sometimes under the driving rain, sometimes under a burning sun, floods of people pass by, flow by, young women holding children in their arms, women who on the way are still giving their breast full of life, full of sap, to keep their babies from crying ... Their skirts are clutched by little children who already know how to walk, superb children, brown-haired and blond, with their curls floating on the breeze; the little girls have big bows in their hair ... And young men, able-bodied A, strong, who do not want to be separated from their families, who prefer to stay with them in the 'work camps' as their fellow citizens in the Germans' pay, who have stayed at home, have solemnly promised them ... And the young women and men who support their exhausted mothers and fathers, sick or bent under the weight of bundles, bags that, when they were embarking the train, they didn't want to give to the men ... who tried to take them, promising they'd find them again in the camp. These are the provisions, changes of clothes for the little ones, a chamber pot for an infant, the saucepan to make him his soup as soon as they arrive, a doll, a toy, these are their poor savings of a whole life. (Vaisman 2005, 43)

Witnessing the arrival of cattle trains and the treatment of the prisoners continually evoked feelings of hatred and rage toward the Nazis. 'It is only hatred that gives us strength, and hope to see the Nazi regime collapse before our eyes, the hope that one day we will help the living world prevent the return of these crimes' (Vaisman 2005, 58). Vaisman was devastated when she witnessed the anguish and helplessness of prisoners who saw their loved ones arriving knowing they were about to die in the gas chambers.

> She [a prisoner] has seen in the line flowing to the crematorium the ones who are dearest to her in the world, the ones who are her reason for being, the ones who gave her the courage to bear her martyr's life. We look on, tense, our teeth clenched in rage; hatred for our executioners makes us tighten our fists, bite our lips. (Vaisman 2005, 54)

---

20 Sima's participation in 'Sport' is evident from her description: "'Sport' meant that under the orders of an SS officer, brandishing a big, heavy stone, they have to walk, run, throw themselves on the ground, get up, jump, crawl on their knees, get up again without stopping, without interruption for an hour and a half, two hours. Blows rain down on the ones who can no longer keep up with the others. And we are in a region that is covered in mud almost all year long. Dirty as pigs, exhausted, dead with fatigue, we return to the block in the evening. And, next morning, work begins again' (Vaisman 2005, 65).

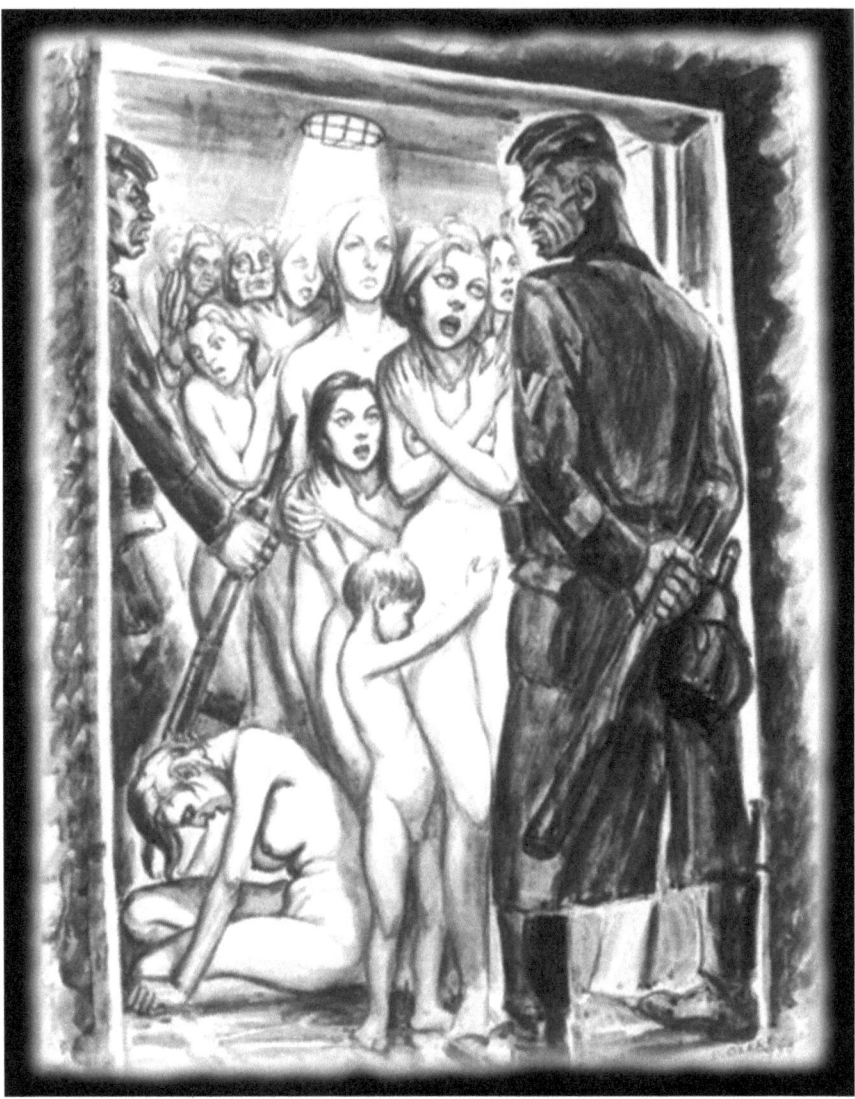

Fig. 3: In the gas chamber.

It is at these times that Vaisman was faced with a dilemma. Should she or the other inmates who knew the fate of the passing wave of the condemned have told them of their fate? She asked what use would rebellion be? Without weapons, their hands empty, they would be defeated in advance. Their action would serve no purpose and their moral and physical torture would only be greater. Sima and her fellow prisoners, stunned and helpless, witnessed the slow procession of these people to the gas chamber. Telling the prisoner of their fate would cause panic and hysteria leading to chaos and bashing, attacks by dogs and execution by shooting. Perversely allowing them to go to their unknown fate arguably was more compassionate, although the artist in this poignant scene, Fig. 3., reveals the fear, hatred, anxiety, defiance and despair of the victims. At the same time the SS guards show contempt and a lack of empathy for the fate of the prisoners. Irrespective Sima was a witness to the gassing and burning of the people: 'אדבוע הווה ידידב'[21] and if they had attempted to warn them of their fate they would have met their death as well. Her description of the fate of children lays bare the inhumanity of the perpetrators.

Fig. 4 is a collage portraying inhumanity at it's worst. In the lower right hand corner Jewish prisoners extracting gold fillings and false teeth from dead Jewish prisoners, victims of the gas chambers. In the center children being shoveled into fire pits or in some cases buried or burnt alive. At the top of the sketch thousands of Jews on their way to the gas chambers and in the left hand corner Jewish women in the delousing chambers. In most of the worst tasks the SS ordered the Kapos and privileged prisoners to do the most heinous tasks.

> The gas chamber has two little windows, barred skylights. Hands cling to them, stretch out to the air, we hear children crying, cries of 'mama, mama,' they call to us for help ... and the room is full (one thousand people in all), two SS, wearing gas masks, approach the two little windows. Pour the gas into them (from cans) and hermetically seal them ... the silence is total. Death takes seven minutes. (Vaisman 2005, 55)

Vaisman's paralysis and powerlessness to prevent the murder of children in the fire pits, the selection of pregnant women for the gas chambers, the images of prisoners seeing their beloved ones innocently heading for the gas chambers and crematoriums is real. Paradoxically, while Vaisman and her colleagues were surrounded by death, life for them continued. In addition to her duties as a block doctor she worked in *Kanada*. Vaisman (2005, 58) recalls her group 'works and eats'.

> The women worked collecting, classifying and packaging all of the belongings of the persons that had arrived [money, clothing, jewellery, blankets, toys, rugs, medicine ... each article in a special bin]. They eat, for they collect the food brought to the camp by the Jews, and either quickly devour what they find or hide the food on their body. (Vaisman 2005, 55)

She is outraged that her colleagues take advantage of those who have been murdered, eating the food collected and laughing and enjoying themselves.

---

21 Holocaust survivors as they are stating that they actually witnessed the atrocity. They are not making it up (Bar-On 2010).

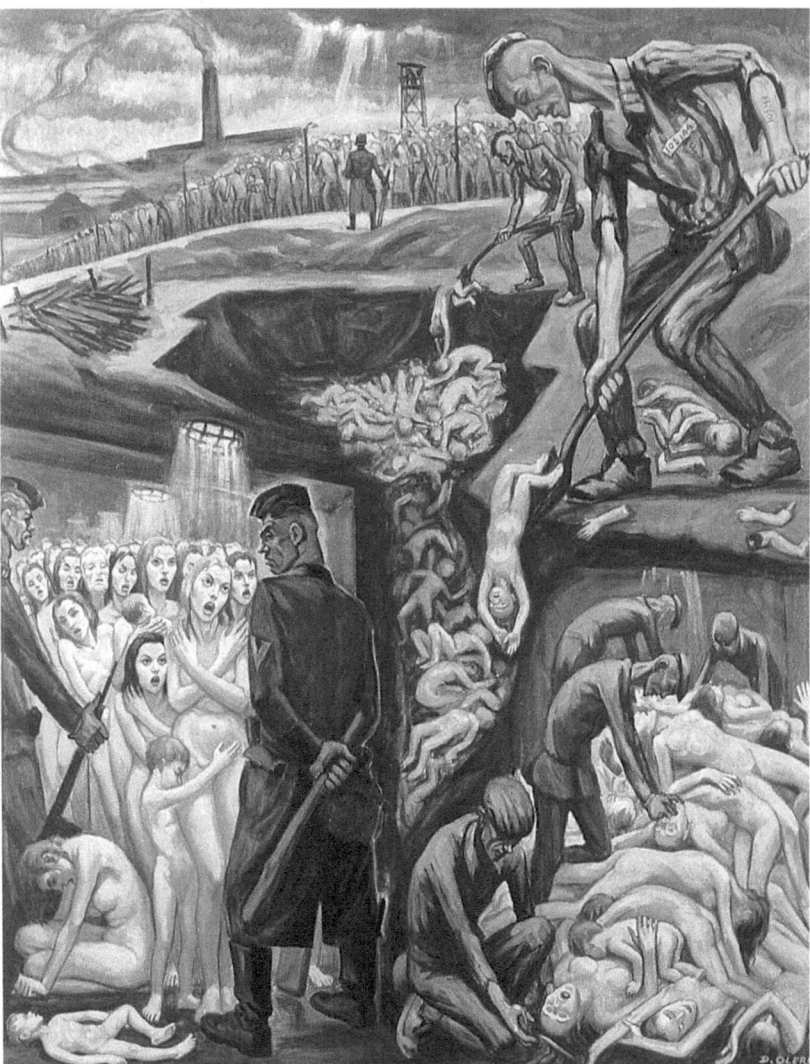

Fig. 4: Inhumanity.

And after twelve hours of work ... these girls, having returned to the block, give themselves veritable orgies of food. What does it matter to them that the flames are rising to the sky, that the stench of scorched bones tightens the throat, that our sisters in misery are withering in pain in the sauna, since the flesh of their flesh has just been torn from them, their children, their mother, their husband, what does it matter that they are already hungry and cold? They eat gluttonously, the fat runs down their fingers, onto the beds, they gossip, they laugh ... No writer, no poet could ever describe this life. Is this what hell is? (Vaisman 2005, 59)

Only a survivor can make judgement. Nevertheless, is Vaisman's outrage directed more at the inhumane and evil conditions in which the prisoners lived rather than the actions of the prisoners who were desperately trying to survive? Under normal conditions these women would have condemned their own behaviour labelling it as outrageous. However, they knew at the first sign of ill health or emaciation they were destined for selection. Under the circumstances the women's actions were normal.

From September 1944 the advance of the Russian army became a reality and plans were made for the evacuation of the camp. This included the liquidation of the prisoner population. It began with the murder of over 4200 Tisanes (gypsies) who were sent to the gas chambers and crematoriums or fire pits. Vaisman notes:

> every night, the headlights from the trucks going to the crematorium ovens light up our windows. We count them during sleepless nights to know how many of our brothers and sisters died that night ... the SS doctor will 'work hard,' he will make selections without stopping. (Vaisman 2005, 62)

Vaisman reveals the perversity of Nazi actions in describing how, with Christmas approaching, pressure was placed on the prisoners to sort and package the hundreds of thousands of items confiscated from prisoners. These were to be sent to Germany as gifts for German families, particularly their children. Despite the impending capitulation of the camp to the advancing Russians, it was business as usual. This included the murder and torture of Jews. She recalls, 'we hear cries for help all night long' (Vaisman 2005, 62). When Vaisman questioned an SS guard on how long it would take to evacuate the camp she replied, 'very quickly – at least 75 per cent will go to the Himmelkommando (the work group in the sky)' (Vaisman 2005, 63). In November 1944, the transports were rare and selections discontinued. Yet the killing continued, '500 children between ten and fourteen years old, still healthy children, children of gypsies they said, coming from Dachau. They were gassed in our camp as soon as they arrived' (Vaisman 2005, 64). On 18 January 1945, the Nazis evacuated the camp and ordered all prisoners to leave on what was to be an arduous seven-day march and train journey in open cars to Ravensbrück[22] and then Neustadt-Glewe. For Vaisman the possibility of surviving Auschwitz evoked cautious hope and relief:

> We don't dare believe we are leaving Brezinki, that they didn't gas all of us, that we are leaving alive. And in weather that's 15 below, we walk cheerfully, quickly, we leave behind

---

22 Ravensbrück, a women's camp was located 50 kilometres north of Berlin. The camp had a capacity for 2000 prisoners; however, over 130,000 prisoners entered through the gates. After the mass exodus from Auschwitz the camp numbers swelled dramatically causing conditions to worsen and mortality rates to climb.

us this cursed land where millions of people lost their lives ... where each one of us has left someone close to us, a parent, a child, a friend. (Vaisman 2005, 66)

The journey from Auschwitz was long and difficult:

We pass in front of all the little camps of Auschwitz. Everything is empty; everywhere fires are burning. And, on the way, we meet other columns of evacuees from Auschwitz, endless columns of women and men, people in rags, scarcely clothed, sick people, beaten out of the hospitals and infirmaries with clubs at the last minute ... We wrap ourselves up in our blankets, support each other and ... we march forward. (Vaisman 2005, 64)

Despite the retreat and the realization that defeat was not far away, the SS culture of terror and death prevailed. The Jews were driven relentlessly and killed when they could not keep up:

We have walked for fourteen hours without stopping, without having a minute of rest ... fatigue began to overtake us. Around midnight, we began to see the corpses of our detainees stretched out in the snow, with a bullet in the head, sometimes in the stomach ... They are the ones, having left before us, who couldn't go any further and were shot down on the way. (Vaisman 2005, 68)

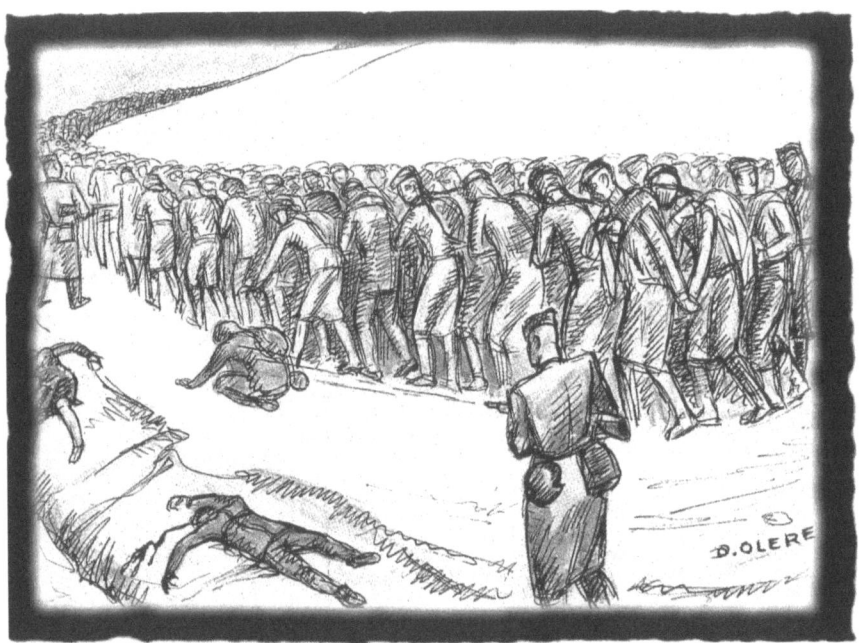

Fig. 5: The Death March. (David Olère, ca. 1945).

Life is made of nothing but steps. More steps, more life, more life, more steps. Each step is a victory over Germany, over the SS, over death, over myself. My companions, known or unknown, stronger or weaker, younger or weaker, women and men, fall and die around me. I must not turn my head to them. It will not help them, it will not help me. When I fall and die, no one will turn his head to me. No one will know. No one will care. But I care. I must survive. I walk and my assignment walks ahead of me. I am able to show, so I must show, so I will show or nobody else will. (Olère & Ohler 1998, 98)

Vaisman and some of her companions thought of escaping, however, they realized their limitations. They did not know the countryside or the language and they had a large Red Cross painted on their backs. From experience in the camp they were fearful and distrusting of the Poles and believed they would be turned away or betrayed. The prisoners were subjected to brutality and immediate death:

With gunshots and blows from clubs, the SS load us up, 100 in each car, and leave us on the track, while they go into the waiting room of the train station ... it is -26 degrees Fahrenheit that night, they say ... the women who died on the way were unloaded onto the road and left there. No one knew their names, or even their numbers. (Vaisman 2005, 69)

On 25 January after seven days marching and travelling on open cattle cars, Vaisman and some two thousand other prisoners arrived at Ravensbrück. Conditions at this camp were similar to Auschwitz. In this new environment Vaisman, with the assistance of a group of doctors and nurses, established a *revier* in the corner of a barrack. Virtually nothing had changed from Auschwitz. Medicines and bandages were almost non-existent, and there was little room for the burgeoning number of sick and injured. The dismissal of all Jewish needs had not subsided. Vaisman (2005, 69) asked the SS Oberschwester (head nurse) for medication for the patients. She replied, 'Aren't you Jewish? You forget that you have no right to live!' On 14 February, Vaisman was sent to Neustadt-Glewe[23] in Mecklenburg where conditions of hardship and loss continued, but with a difference. Not only were the Jewish prisoners subject to abuse by the German SS, in addition the non-Jewish German and Polish women prisoners beat and bullied the Jews whenever possible. The abuse was relentless:

Every day, we stand outside for hours at rollcall. After rollcall, they distribute bread to us, the ration already diminished to a sixth. After the third day we're given a little soup, three or four spoonfuls per person. But each time after this distribution and this roll-call, we have to return to the barn under blows that rain down and, inside, more blows await us, from Polish and German women defending their places. We are beaten to make us leave the barn,

---

23 Sub-camp of Ravensbrück. A camp for women from mid 1944 until May 1945.

beaten to make us return to it, beaten to go to the toilet (no water this whole time), beaten for having moved a little. (Vaisman 2005, 73)

The misery never stopped for Vaisman, yet after three concentration camps (excluding Drancy) she kept going. She held strong. In Neustadt-Glewe, Jewish women were not permitted to work as doctors in the infirmaries. However, this did not prevent Vaisman from continuing her work with patients. She carried out prophylactic (precautionary) sanitary work in the blocks keeping scabies and lice under control, found or organized[24] medicine for as many patients as possible, and took the sickest to the hospital. On 3 May 1945, the Russian army liberated the camp and Vaisman was free '... the Russians ... supplied us wonderfully with provisions – milk, butter, meat every day, potatoes, sugar. They dressed us, gave us cloth and seamstresses to make clothes for our patients. They gave us leather and shoemakers to have sandals made for us' (Vaisman 2005, 68). After approximately seven weeks, most of her previously sick and weak patients had regained sufficient strength to be repatriated to their country of origin or moved to refugee centres. Vaisman's epic journey was arguably one of the most courageous of all survivors. She lived in the worst camp, Birkenau, for the entire period of incarceration of approximately 12 months. She lived and worked with the prisoners, without respite. Her memoirs reveal little of her emotions except for outrage at the atrocities. She concentrated on the conditions and suffering of her fellow prisoners.

She appeared to be leading a double life. It was that of a person holding her personal pain inside, yet at the same time, she was a person who endured and witnessed emotional, psychological and physical pain and suffering that defies description. Sima returned to Paris. She was in poor health and weak, weighing less than thirty kilograms (less than seventy pounds). According to her nephew Emanuel Marom, she was so malnourished that she was unrecognizable to either friends or family. However, with the support of her friends, particularly her cousin Abram Neiman and his wife Emma, Sima regained her strength and health. In 1947, she went to Bucharest to visit her mother and sister, both of whom had escaped the camps. Yet even this journey was beset with difficulties. She still had Romanian citizenship at the time and the authorities would not allow her to leave Romania to return to Paris. Through the help of French friends, former resistance members, she was eventually able to return to Paris. Upon returning to Paris Sima became a French citizen and settled in Paris renting a small apartment near Porte de St Cloud, one room of which she converted into a dentist's practice. With her diverse interests, including politics, literature, music and art, she shared her life with family and friends from all walks of life. It was these people who were most

---

24 This term was a euphuism for stealing.

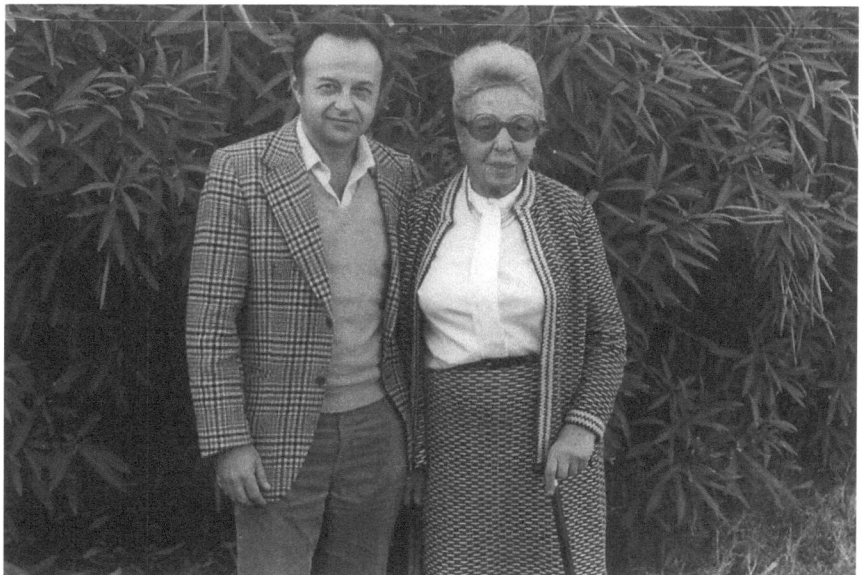

Fig. 6: Sima with nephew Emanuel Maroon after the war. (courtesy of Sima Vaisman's extended family and friends).

important to her. As her nephew wrote, 'She was the glue that kept the various members of the family and friends in contact and had patience for every one of them' (Marom 2011). According to her nephews and nieces their aunt 'had integrity and was blessed with a high sense of morality and professional ethics.'

Her decision to record her experiences as soon as possible after Auschwitz is testimony to Vaisman's determination to bear witness to what happened and to reveal the full extent of the evil committed by the Germans. Her rage and hatred towards the Germans continued well after Auschwitz. According to Emanuel, photographed with Sima in Fig. 6., she never set foot in Germany and initially refused to accept reparations from the German Government. She later accepted payments in order to establish an annual grant for medical students from Tel Aviv University to study abroad. She wanted to give back to medicine as she felt that medicine had saved her life in Auschwitz-Birkenau. Sima Vaisman, as was the case of most Jewish doctors who worked in the death and labour camps, was an ordinary person who was called upon to do extraordinary acts that helped and comforted fellow prisoners under the most horrendous conditions. After the war Sima continued in the field of health. In the camps, she witnessed evil and inhumanity and after the war she could witness and take comfort in the results of her own acts of goodness that contributed to humanity.

Dr Vaisman passed away in Paris on 31 May 1997 at the age of 95.

2 Louis Micheels

They [the SS] loved to delegate limited power to a
select few, for whom it became a vehicle of survival.
Louis Micheels (1989, 54)

Louis Micheels was born on 6 June 1917 in the picturesque and prosperous village of Bloemendaal, some eighteen miles from Amsterdam. Louis lived with his parents Clara and Albert, older sister Elf, brother Lex, and their servants. They resided in a large Tudor-style home in what he describes as 'an enclave where I had been shielded from most forms of physical or emotional deprivation' (Micheels 1989, 6). He came from a privileged family as he and his brother and sister had a nanny. When he was three years old, the intensity of his relationship with his nanny Joop made his mother dismiss her in the belief their relationship was unhealthily close. Louis does not discuss further this matter other than to confess he felt her loss keenly and years later took up regular correspondence with Joop.

Nevertheless, Louis remembers his childhood as a very happy time. He was close to his brother, Lex and sister, Elf and they grew up doing what normal kids for their age did and enjoyed. From a very early age Louis formed close bonds with others. The Micheels' family life was very stable and ordered. Louis' father Albert was a successful broker in Amsterdam whose hobby was collecting antique furniture and paintings. Micheels describes him as a kind disciplinarian who was passionate about sport and staying fit. Encouraged by his father he too thrived on sport and exercise; something which he later saw as having given him a toughness and resilience that stood him in good stead. Louis' mother Clara was a devoted wife and loving mother. Emphasis was placed on education and the children were encouraged to work hard at school. Although Micheels was bright, he did not enjoy the heavy workload and high standards expected of students at his school, the elite Het Stedelijk Gymnasium, in Haarlem. He studied French and German, becoming proficient in both, and learned to play the cello. The ability to speak several languages was of benefit in the camps and often was life-saving. In their leisure time the family went hiking, bicycling and sailing together. Louis also became an avid equestrian.

The family considered themselves Conservative rather than Orthodox Jews. The family was not observant although Albert attended synagogue regularly and he encouraged and expected Louis to do likewise. Louis had both Jewish and non-Jewish friends and his family would celebrate St Nicholas with Christian friends while these same friends celebrated Chanukah with the Micheels. At no

https://doi.org/10.1515/9783110598216-005

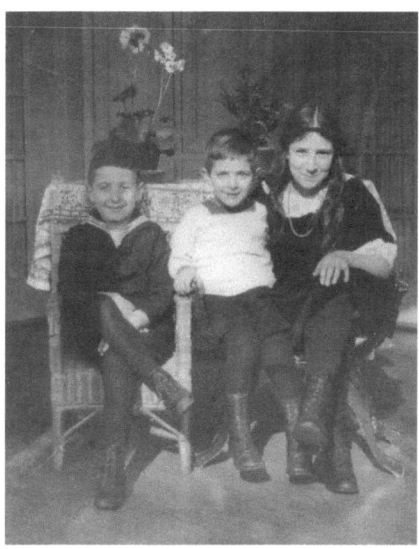

Fig. 7: Micheels with older sister Elf and younger brother Lex, in Bloemendaal. (Courtesy of the Micheels' family)

time prior to the invasion of Holland did Louis feel touched or threatened by antisemitism.

In 1938, Micheels commenced medical studies at the University of Utrecht where he shared a flat with Anton, a non-Jewish friend who was also studying medicine. He found life as a student exciting and challenging and enjoyed the friendships and camaraderie with his fellow students. He joined the student union Het Utrechtsch Studenten Corps and a Zionist student group. It was at a meeting of the Zionist group in 1939 that he met and fell in love with Nora, a music student from Amsterdam. He recalls the wonderful time he and Nora spent together in the beginning of their relationship, 'walking in the dunes, enjoying the burgeoning spring, the flowers, the smell of jasmine, the countryside' (Micheels 1989, 17). Nora was to become central to his life for the next six to seven years until the end of the war.

Despite Louis and Nora leading a rather carefree existence, the people of Holland were increasingly aware of and alarmed by the changes occurring in Germany with the coming to power of Adolf Hitler and the implementation of his policies and actions towards Jews. In 1939 with the invasion of Poland and the rumours of harsh measures against the Jews in Germany, Austria and Poland, Micheels became anxious that conflict could break out between Germany and Holland. In 1940 his fears were confirmed and realizing his family was in grave danger decided they must escape their homeland. Neither his brother nor sister still lived in Holland. His brother had fled to France and from there migrated to New York. His sister had married an Englishman

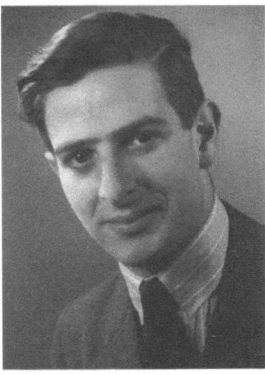

Fig. 8: Micheels as a medical student before the war. (courtesy of the Micheels' family)

in 1934 and migrated to Australia. Micheels felt responsible for the safety of his parents. He persuaded them to travel to Ijmuiden and escape by ship to England. However, on seeing the huge number of Jews who had descended on Ijmuiden hoping to escape, his parents lost heart and returned home to Bloemendaal.

After minimal resistance from the Dutch forces the Nazis took control of the country in May 1940. To Micheels' surprise, initially life under Nazi occupation was not threatening, and there existed an almost holiday-like atmosphere. The people were assured that life would become normal again. Shops re-opened for business. His father resumed work. Micheels returned to university and enjoyed hiking, swimming and sailing with Nora and his friends. Nora had become an important part of his life and they spoke of getting married. However, despite the apparent normality of life, Micheels was aware of what was rumoured to be taking place in other Nazi-occupied countries. He believed that life for Jews in Holland would change for the worse. By late 1940 and early 1941 changes were taking place. Dutch Nazis in their black uniforms, German troops and SS officers marching through the streets of both Amsterdam and rural districts became a common sight.

Micheels' father lost his business and the family home was repossessed. The family was forced to move from Bloemendaal to Amsterdam where they lived in a house with several other families. Still Micheels' parents refused to listen to his pleas for the family to go into hiding or escape as Micheels describes,

> ...He [Albert] did not want to burden or endanger others. Deeper down, he must have felt like giving up, as if the strain was becoming unbearable. My mother seemed even more depressed and less able to act. They reflected a general mood of surrender, as if the end could not come too soon. (Micheels 1989, 6)

Louis' father and mother were typical of many older people who did not understand or accept the reality that Hitler was determined to carry out his plans to exterminate the Jews of Europe. His parents refused to leave their cherished homeland and as was the case of many aged people considered themselves too old to start over again in a new country. Despite the decision by his parents Micheels and Nora decided to flee Holland but were betrayed and arrested by the Dutch Nazis. In November 1942, they were transported to Mechelen[25] transit camp, Belgium, where they were imprisoned for a further six months. It was in Mechelen that Micheels learned important lessons on how to survive the Nazi camp environment with 'my basic drive for survival my only weapon' (Micheels 1989, 6). Carl, a prisoner of Polish-German descent who he befriended, insisted that obedience to SS or Kapo orders was critical to survival. Carl maintained that it was essential to 'play their game' (Micheels 1989, 6) and that in doing so he could get into the levels of the camp society where the power and the food were. Micheels strictly adhered to this rule throughout his time in Auschwitz. He either consciously or unconsciously would attempt to go unnoticed, obey SS and Kapo[26] orders and form friendships with prisoners of influence. As soon as he was confronted with a toxic situation such as assignment to a block with a sadistic Kapo, he would work to be transferred.

In Mechelen, Micheels learnt there was no human value system:

> In this sort of camp our customary system of values had almost ceased to exist, and with it the possibility of uniting the prison population against the oppressor. In the camp people were useless. The only purpose of their existence was to serve the oppressor's sadistic needs. (Micheels 1989, 53)

He also realized that to survive, it was every person for himself. This understanding influenced his further decisions in the prison camps. When Micheels and Nora were in Mechelen, he and Henk, another Jewish doctor twenty years his senior, were advised that one of them would be transported to the east, usually a death camp such as Auschwitz. The other would remain in Mechelen as camp doctor. Micheels was chosen to stay. Henk pleaded for Micheels to go in his place, arguing that

---

25 The Mechelen transit camp, officially SS-Sammellager Mecheln in German, was a detention and deportation camp established in the former Dossin Barracks at Mechelen in German-occupied Belgium. The transit camp was run by the Sicherheitspolizei (SiPo-SD), a branch of the SS-Reichssicherheitshauptamt, in order to collect and deport Jews and other minorities such as Romani mainly out of Belgium towards the labor camp of Heydebreck-Cosel and the concentration camps of Auschwitz-Birkenau in German occupied Poland.
26 Kapos were trustee inmates who were appointed by the SS to supervise the other prisoners. Their status as 'Prominente', which afforded them certain privileges, also required them to be harsh and cruel with the prisoners. Some were Jewish.

being so much older and having a wife and three young children he did not stand a chance of survival. Nora and Micheels were young and strong enough to make it, but Micheels (1989, 57) would not be swayed and refused to relent to Henk's pleas. Although they were not married, the bond between the two lovers was a defining factor in Micheels' life in the camps. He relied on Nora for emotional support and the motivation to survive. The first sign of his dependency on Nora occurred in Mechelen when Louis was accused of being a homosexual and attacked by a number of Jews, 'punched, cursed at and pushed down the stairs' (Micheels 1989, 55). He recalls he felt 'humiliated, helpless and enraged. I ran back to Nora in our dorm, unable to hold back my tears' (Micheels 1989, 55). Again he expressed his reliance on Nora when the appalling conditions they were experiencing had led Louis to feel that they had reached 'what seemed the nadir of our existence' and that, 'if it had not been for Nora ... we would not have survived much longer' (Micheels 1989, 56).

On 18 April, 1943 Micheels and Nora joined the twentieth RSHA transport from Belgium to Auschwitz arriving at the camp on April 22 with 1400 other Jews (Czech 1990, 381).[27] According to Micheels upon arrival he met Dr Eduard Wirths,[28] the head medical officer of the camp. Micheels explained to Wirths he was a doctor and was in charge of the transport that had just arrived. Wirths told him 'to contact him (Wirths) later at the camp, and that we (Nora and Louis) would be well taken care of' (Micheels 1989, 65). At the ramp they were selected to go right to the labour camp. Micheels was sent to Monowitz and Nora sent to the main camp to work as a nurse in Block 10, the infamous women's medical experimentation Block.

Separated from Nora and alone in 'the selfish, impersonal atmosphere', he had a sense of 'being nothing' (Micheels 1989, 68). It was in this state that he underwent the initiation process of being shaved, showered, tattooed and provided with an odd assortment of clothing (Micheels 1989, 66). Being tattooed [No 117641] was a profoundly disturbing experience for Louis and an indicator of the seriousness of his predicament:

> Not only was a bodily change being imposed on me, but [it was] an irrevocable, irreversible one. It dawned on me that this camp was far more dangerous than either Mechelen or St Gillies and that I was probably not meant to come out alive. Still, I did not give up hope. (Micheels 1989, 67)

---

27 From a transport of 2,800 men, women and children from Greece, only 255 men and 413 women were selected for work; the remaining 2,132 were killed in the gas chambers. Thus over 3,000 Jews were murdered on that day alone. Approximately 25,000 Jews were sent to Auschwitz from Mechelen, of which only 1,240 survived (Kazerne Dossin n.d.)

28 Wirths was the Chief SS doctor (SS-Standortarzt) at the Auschwitz concentration camp from September 1942 to January 1945. Thus, Wirths had formal responsibility for everything undertaken by the nearly 20 SS doctors (including Josef Mengele, Horst and Carl) who worked in the medical sections of Auschwitz between 1942–1945.

He worked in the labour gangs for several days. In a perverse sort of way, this was a blessing. He saw the weak, exhausted, brutalized, and emaciated physical state of his fellow prisoners. He realized that he could not survive such conditions for long. He knew that to survive the camp he needed to find work that did not involve heavy labour or work exposed to the elements of severe cold or heat. Such an opportunity arose when the SS were looking for doctors to work in the Reviers and hospitals. Louis and his friend Albert, his travelling companion, commenced work as nurses in one of the barracks of the hospital in Monowitz, Auschwitz III. Louis was optimistic, 'I told Albert that I believed this assignment would save our lives. He did not seem convinced, but I was ... In this situation, I saw some hope of surviving' (Micheels 1989, 68). Within a very short time, conditions improved dramatically for Micheels. He worked in an environment far removed from that which he had left. The prisoner doctor, a non-Jew, was friendly, caring and experienced in camp life and the conditions were better.

> There was none of the rigid drill atmosphere of the rest of the camp, in which even bodies of inmates who had died while working had to be carried to roll call. Our food was also superior. We got at least two bowls of soup and frequently a sort of farina as well ... sometimes during the day we could sneak in a brief nap, an unbelievable luxury. Strange as it may seem, the future was beginning to look a little less bleak. (Micheels 1989, 70)

Louis worked in the camp hospital for three weeks where he contracted a sore throat and a fever. It was forbidden to keep any prisoners with infectious diseases at industrial and manufacturing sites. After being diagnosed with diphtheria by a fellow Jewish doctor, Samuel, he was sent to the Krankenhaus (Hospital) in Auschwitz I (Stammlager). He was on a truck that was taking several dead bodies to the crematoria, and the driver made a detour and dropped him off at the Stammlager, where he was treated in an isolation area. Louis believed this to be luck, however, it is unlikely the driver would have acted without authority. While in hospital Louis received a letter from Nora:

> I am in the same camp as you, only a few hundred feet away in a special block, number 10. Albert was transferred from Buna to here shortly after you. He saw you by chance when you looked out of a window. Sonya is also here. Both of us are nurses taking care of the women who are used for experiments from which Sonya and I as nurses are exempted. Albert helps bring the soup from the kitchen to us, and has talked with Sonya. I hope you feel better. Write me soon. David will get it to me. Love, hugs and kisses, Nora. (Micheels 1989, 75)

Knowing Nora was alive gave Louis hope, 'It should not be difficult to imagine how this dramatic turn of events made me feel. I could see some possibility of survival, something and somebody to live for' (Micheels 1989, 76). Here Micheels exposed his insecurity and belief that as long as he had contact with Nora he had a chance of survival. It can be argued he was in denial, for after all he was in a death camp and his belief that Nora in some way was going to be his saviour was unrealistic. But it was an example of the power of hope that solidified the will to live. After three weeks he recovered and was assigned to the camp hospital of the Stammlager. His experience in the hospital was horrendous.

> Temporarily, at least, I had to sleep in the same ward as the patients. Several double bunks, one above the other, had been set-aside in the corner for us. To my dismay I discovered that my bunk, like most of the others, was infested with fleas. After one night I was covered with flea bites. A few days later I found some flea powder; it helped but did not solve the problem. One had to be careful not to scratch: the danger of infection was great ... They were thin to the point of emaciation and given to paroxysms of coughing and suffocating intensively. Some hardly touched their food. I tried feeding them but with limited success. Ben, a young Dutch Jew, was so far gone that he did not even want his little portion of bread ... Ben had given up; he did not want to live. (Micheels 1989, 80)

Evidence of prisoners' desperation to survive was often found in the hospitals and infirmaries. Micheels recalled the behaviour of such prisoners that turned them into savage animals. The hospitals for the Jewish prisoners were a paradox for in one sense they were the anti-chamber for selection to phenol injection or the gas chambers or they were fertile ground for prisoners to scavenge food and clothing from dying patients. He referred to Ben, who was close to death:

> I noticed that other patients, seeing his condition, his abdication of life, had their eyes on his bread and soup. Stealing bread was the worst crime anyone could commit punished by often fatal beatings ... The step from human being to savage animal was but a small one. Yet those unable to avoid such a metamorphosis often could not survive. Therefore, a close friendship where the human qualities and values could be preserved in a small enclave, took on enormous importance. Such a bond was essential as a protection against losing all traces of civilized behaviour, and with them a true sense of hope and reason for survival. (Micheels 1989, 80)

It appears that Micheels at this stage of his life in Auschwitz recognized the need to cling to some form of humanity. His subsequent actions led me to conclude he realized the importance of relationships that provided him with some sense of civilized normality. At the same time altruism gave him self-esteem and a sense of goodness and dignity. Although he was concerned about working in the tuberculosis ward, his position as doctor-nurse immediately benefited his status in the camp: 'I realized I was sort of upper-middle-class in the camp society' (Micheels 1989, 84). Micheels reveals little of his work although he recalls cases of individuals he helped, such as Dirk, whom he knew from Mechelen. Dirk was suffering from a badly infected foot that was not responding to treatment. He would try and lift his spirits and take him extra soup or bread but his efforts were to no avail and he was selected for the gas chamber. Micheels recalls that when he became aware that a selection was to take place, he would conceal case records or send those patients with little chance of passing the test to the bathroom or another hiding place so that 'In this way, even if we could not do very much, they perhaps had a chance of survival, or at least could die a natural death' (Micheels 1989, 87).

From his oral testimony, it is clear that Micheels' worked with Samuel at the Stammlager, assisting him with operations. Neither in his memoir nor in his testimony does he refer to taking part in human experiments or divulge what type of operations he assisted with. He never worked in Block 10 or for Clauberg,[29] but it is possible that he was involved in the operations Samuel performed in the sterilization programs. To Micheels' consternation Samuel suddenly disappeared, assumed murdered by the SS after which he was then transferred to Block 12. The move to this block is interesting for Block 12 is where operations took place to castrate men and perform operations on women to remove the uterus. Samuel's sudden disappearance and his own impending move filled Micheels with anxiety and fear 'Even though I had developed certain immunity to living in the shadow of death, events like this were a shock and threatened to shatter the tenuous structure of relative security I had erected' (Micheels 1989, 85).

From the beginning of his incarceration, despite the conditions and atmosphere, Micheels was hopeful he could overcome most challenges. His family stated he was an optimistic and very positive person. The lesson he had learned in Mechelen of the importance of going unnoticed became a hallmark of his existence. But Micheels had fears that he believed if not appeased could be the end for him. His dread was the loss of his status as a privileged prisoner, resulting in his return to the labour gangs and his loss of contact with Nora:

> My contact with Nora was without doubt the cornerstone of that security ... the idea of being separated from Nora was more than I could bear. I could not believe it; I knew this would be the end of me. (Micheels 1989, 90)

Micheels moved to a new block that provided him with better conditions and a safer environment 'in a clean environment, in-doors, decently fed and away from the dangers of tuberculosis' (Micheels 1989, 92). His responsibilities were to keep

---

29 Clauberg conducted human experiments in Auschwitz mainly in the infamous Block 10. After gaining his medical degree with a specialty in gynaecology he commenced research on female fertility hormones and their application in infertility treatments. He was appointed by Himmler in December 1942 to carry out research in Auschwitz to sterilize women on mass. He offered a cheap and easy way by injecting formaldehyde preparations into their uteruses – without anaesthetics – The guinea pigs, mainly young Greek Jewish women either died or suffered permanent damage.

the barracks of SS guards spotlessly clean and tidy. He found the guards whose rooms he cleaned would leave bread or 'come by with a container of pureed potatoes or cereal, part of their regular meal' (Micheels 1989, 92). Micheels was essentially his own boss in that he could work at his own pace as long as the job was done. Most importantly, he was still able to have almost daily contact with Nora. In January 1944, the Gestapo accused him of having contact with and working for the Dutch underground. Louis' instincts urged him to find a new place of work. He secured work at the Hygiene Institute of the Waffen-SS Raisko[30] through his friend Dorus. A vacancy existed in the 'matrix kitchen,' where they prepared extracts, chemical additives for agar plates, and food bases for their bacteriological cultures. His work place was modern, clean and air-conditioned, and he worked with a congenial group of Jews and non-Jews that included Dorus and Ellis, his best friends apart from Nora. The friends accompanied each other to and from work every morning and evening, but their daily trip was a constant reminder of the paradox of their situation and the fragility of their existence.

> The laboratory was four miles from the camp and it took us about an hour to walk there. But it was a pleasant walk, at least if the weather was not too bad, along the banks of the Solar river, past an agricultural station staffed by women prisoners, to whom we waved enthusiastically in passing ... in the distance, we could see the chimneys of the crematorium in Birkenau. It was a glaring and dramatic contrast: on one side the beauty of nature, on the other the horror of the worst mass murder of all times ... the contrast intensified the feeling of impending danger. (Micheels 1989, 100)

Despite Micheels working so far from the main camp, he and Nora managed to see each other regularly though not as frequently as before. He felt a desperate need,

---

30 The Institute of Hygiene had been headquartered in the concentration camp Auschwitz I until spring 1943 when it was relocated to a place called Raisko, five kilometers away from Auschwitz. The activities of the Institute of Hygiene centered on medical analysis for the SS, the Wehrmacht, the police force, and the concentration camp (including Joseph Mengele, the doctor notorious for his experiments on humans). Laboratory examinations from the Institute of Hygiene included samples of urine, blood, stool, sputum, and throat swabs. The documents from the Institute in the collection of the archive contain approximately 40,000 les from the period between April 10, 1943 and January 12, 1945, of which nine volumes are general ledgers, eight volumes are subsidiary ledgers, and the rest of the papers are arranged in sixty-two folders. The documents allow for insights into the inner workings of the Institute of Hygiene. They include notes about treated prisoners of Auschwitz and its satellite camps as well as members of the SS troops stationed at Auschwitz. Frequently, these documents have turned out to be the only written record remaining about prisoners. Beyond that, there is also information about members of the administrative ranks of the Institute of Hygiene of the Waffen-SS and prisoners employed there as aides. Furthermore, the documents contain detailed lists of materials and devices ordered by the Institute of Hygiene of the Waffen-SS (Kozub 2009).

both physical and emotional, to see Nora. Strangely, on Sundays they would meet to have a sort of brunch, almost a feast, with some of the delicacies from the package from Holland, as Louis describes,

> It is almost impossible to describe how much these visits meant to me. To be actually close to Nora, to touch her hand, to kiss her ... to daydream about returning home, to eat together – was the greatest source of strength. (Micheels 1989, 106)

Even under the threat of being caught and punished, he had a habit of passing by Nora's window every morning:

> ... Just before starting on the trek to Raisko, and throw[ing] a stick or stone against the screen to announce my presence ... just seeing her to start the day was so important for me that on the few occasions I could not see her I felt deprived of something essential. I would feel less human, like a cipher, living in a world of greyness with neither light nor shadow. (Micheels 1989, 106)

In his new work place, he encountered SS Untersturmführer Hans Münch,[31] an SS doctor. According to Louis, Münch was 'friendly, showed personal interest in people, never deliberately humiliated anybody' and thus seemed 'oddly out of place in the SS' (Micheels 1989, 101). Münch was to prove a significant ally. While working at the institute, Micheels suffered appendicitis. A Polish doctor, Boris, carried out the appendectomy, but it was Münch who helped him convalesce after the operation and allowed him to keep in daily contact with Nora. Micheels felt immense relief and gratitude: 'Nora's presence here was miraculous: a woman in, of all places, a male hospital ward in Auschwitz. To touch her, to feel her hand, her kiss, gave me the kind of strength I needed to pull through' (Micheels 1989, 101). However, although conditions at Raisko were relatively good, Micheels was afraid. He was subject to personal humiliation and threats by SS Hauptsturmführer Bruno Weber, the SS doctor who was head of the institute. Weber was demanding, vicious and arrogant. He often tested Micheels, who knew that any error of judgment on his part could be

---

31 Hans Münch became a controversial figure after the war. He was a SS physician assigned to Auschwitz and carried out bacteriological research at the research institute at Rosko. It was compulsory for every SS doctor to take part in selections at the rail ramps. After participating in a number he refused to continue and this was permitted. A number of prisoners including Micheels came to his defence at his trial for war crimes at the Auschwitz trials in 1947. He was the only prisoner acquitted. Later, he returned to Germany and worked as a practising physician in Roßhaupten in Bavaria. In later life he made comments in interviews that suggest he agreed with the exterminations that took place and gave justification for the death of prisoners during human experiments. The German government commenced legal action against him but did not proceed due to his mental health.

disastrous. With the exception of Münch, all personnel in charge of the institute were typical Nazis, anti-Semitic, mean and brutal. One was an Austrian, sergeant Zabel, who according to Micheels had the dangerous look of somebody out for revenge. Consequently, Micheels made every effort to be inconspicuous. Although Block 10 could only be accessed by authorized personnel Münch was able to arrange permission for the prisoners to take packages into the block and Micheels was regularly able to visit Nora. Micheels was devastated when on one occasion he was not given a package, and despite his appeals to Münch, he was not able to go and see Nora.

> I do not believe that I had ever before felt quite so helpless. Unable to hold back tears, I told Dorus what had happened … I felt that the rug was being pulled out from under me and I was again confronted with the precarious nature of my existence. (Micheels 1989, 108)

From mid-1944 the constant sound of far off Russian guns indicated the camp would soon be liberated. Micheels, however, had developed peritonitis and feared that he would not recover in time for the liberation. During this period Nora had been sent to a block that was outside the camp, and Micheels did not see her again until after the war. On 17 January 1945 without forewarning the Nazis ordered the camp to be evacuated. Micheels and the prisoner population commenced the infamous Death March. He recalls that he felt a sense of hope and was excited at the prospect of leaving Auschwitz. He also felt apprehension. After his experiences with the Nazis, he was unsure what would ultimately be their fate, but knew of the possibility that they would be executed. Fortunately, being a 'privileged' prisoner Micheels had access to better provisions:

> I had a pair of good shoes and a pair of well-fitting galoshes over them, so my feet were warm and dry. I also had a pair of warm woolen [sic] mittens that Nora had knitted for me just a few days before, and a woolen [sic] headband over my ears. (Micheels 1989, 129)

From Auschwitz to Dachau, their final destination, the journey by foot and cattle train took ten days. The conditions were atrocious. Beatings and killing continued unabated. For three days, they marched approximately fifty miles through the bitter cold with little clothing and virtually no food. The excitement and even enthusiasm felt by Micheels at the start of the march soon vanished as the SS vented their anger and impatience on the prisoners who were lagging behind. Their orders were to shoot any prisoner who could not continue, so prisoners who fell or stumbled were shot. Louis aware of his surroundings did not dare to sit down during rest periods in fear of not being able to get up again and executed. Micheels believed that before the trip had ended all prisoners would meet their end. After a train journey of one and a half days they arrived at Breslau and after another trip on foot they arrived at Gross Rosen. It was 22 January 1945. The conditions at Gross Rosen were similar to those in Auschwitz. To Micheels consternation he was no longer considered a privileged prisoner and received the same treatment as all prisoners:

> We were packed in like sardines. Later, when things calmed down a bit, we each had a couple of square feet to sit down in. Thirst began to bother most of us, including me. The salty hash was having its effects. Up until then I had not known that thirst could be even worse than hunger. We could not get out to the washroom in the adjoining barracks; besides there was no water. (Micheels 1989, 135)

The final part of the journey was once again in an open railroad car and ended in Dachau, Bavaria as Louis recalls:

> There was a definite crescendo of horror and cruelty on this journey. We travelled for days on end, frequently standing still under the watchful eyes of the omnipresent SS guards. We received food, some watery soup, only once, when we stopped at a station. We kept each other warm by huddling close ... we were all starving, and I seriously thought that if worst came to worst I could always kill myself by jumping out of the train and being shot, but I had not reached that point. (Micheels 1989, 135)

At Dachau conditions for Micheels and other members of the Hygiene Institute were greatly improved. The camp was in the middle of a typhus epidemic, and Louis and other Jewish doctors were instructed to set up a new lab in the camp hospital. They received better living conditions and received food packages. To Micheels' anguish however, when there was some glimmer of hope, orders came through that several hundred prisoners including Micheels' group were to be transferred to a labour camp. After intervention by Clauberg the members of the Raisko group were told they would stay. It was 'as if by a miracle, we were saved and taken to a block that was unusually clean and un-crowded' (Micheels 1989, 138). Micheels was overwhelmed with the conditions of his new surroundings and considered he was living in luxury compared to life in Auschwitz.

Still, Micheels missed Nora and worried about her fate. Yet he realized that he had survived the harshest and most frightful experience without Nora. Micheels throughout his incarceration believed Nora was his lifeline and gave him the will to live. Yet in the end he realized he could survive without Nora. At the same time, it becomes obvious that Micheels needed the company of others and he befriended many prisoners, doctors and fellow workers. It became a coping mechanism whereby he put his energy into human relations.

On 1 May 1945 Louis was free and re-entered the world he had left behind in November 1942:

> so very long ago, a world with which, except for a few precious moments, we had had no direct or tangible connection for years, and to which there had been only the faintest chance

> of ever returning. Now that this chance had materialized, I was in a daze… Very slowly I began to realize that I was actually free, my own master, once again a real person who did not need to fear that any moment may be the last. (Micheels 1989, 154)

His first days of freedom were in the town of Mittenwald, Germany, and his next journey was to take him to displaced persons' camps (DP) from Mittenwald to Mannheim and to Paris. In the DP camps conditions were poor with many ex-prisoners suffering from typhoid and lice. With his colleagues, Micheels established clinics and emergency rooms for the sick and weak. He worked in these centres until he was sent to the next DP camp. In Paris he was offered and accepted a paid position by the chief medical doctor of the Dutch government based in Paris:

> He offered us a paid job, room and board included, as his assistants. In view of the bad situation in Holland we decided to accept, especially since he told us that we could accompany weekly transports of patients being repatriated to Holland. (Micheels 1989, 165)

Nora was constantly on his mind, and hoping she was still alive Louis longed to return to Holland. He discovered Nora was in Amsterdam. On June 6, Micheels accompanying sick patients back home, arrived in Holland and journeyed to the city. Unfortunately, Nora had changed and told him that her feelings were now different and she wanted their relationship, as they knew it, to end. Micheels was upset to lose Nora on whom he had depended during their incarceration. Yet he was determined to overcome this heavy loss, and he recalls in his memoirs that he reverted to the experiences and tools that had been so important for his survival in Auschwitz. In Auschwitz he reached out to friends, he tried to stay positive and he kept occupied. Now that he was home, he was determined to stay active and he planned a future that involved furthering his medical studies and starting a new life in America, close to his family. What he had gone through had given him a greater appreciation of life:

> My heightened sense of freedom and appreciation of life in general combined with an intense hunger to savour it fully helped me to overcome the painful wound. (Micheels 1989, 179)

His actions and behaviour showed his resilience, a trait that was present throughout his imprisonment, the Death March and now his break up with Nora. His will to live never left him and he used this customary strategy to endure. He called on his friends who loved him and gave him companionship. Nora was a lifeline for him during his worst moments. His ability to get through intolerable situations, particularly after Auschwitz, is testimony to his courage and hardiness. He migrated to the US, married Ina and thereafter Elizabeth and Ron were born. A new phase in Micheels professional life was also born. The photo below shows Micheels as a rather young

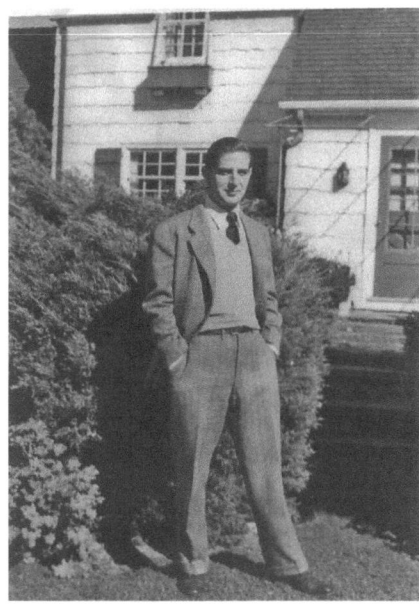

Fig. 9: Dr. Micheels in the US after the Holocaust.
(courtesy of the Micheels' family)

confident man who according to his family was a practicing psychiatrist. The handsome smiling face was hiding a life of unbearable suffering and adversity.

After graduating from medical school and working in a clinical practice he entered the world of academia lecturing in the medical faculty of Yale University. He subsequently became Associate Clinical Professor specialising in teaching medical students how to communicate with patients. Micheels continued both his private practice and teaching at Yale until 2002 when, at the age of 85, he retired.

During the early years of Micheels' life in Bloemendaal, he and his family were very active in sport and outdoor activities such as hiking, sailing and horse riding. After the war and once settled in America, Micheels continued an active life, sailing his own boat, a thirty-foot Atlantic class sailboat that he raced with his wife and children. He stopped sailing in 1988 at the age of eighty-nine. In addition to his active sporting life, from 1990 he took up woodwork as a hobby building furniture. While his father had collected furniture, Micheels made it.

Louis Micheels led a full life tempered by hardship, loss and tragedy. Yet he survived to become a husband, father, grandfather, doctor and teacher. Unlike the thousands of Jewish doctors who did not survive the labour and death camps, Micheels had the opportunity to contribute to humanity as a carer and teacher.

Louis Micheels died on 6 June 2008 at the age of 91. Ina died in 2011.

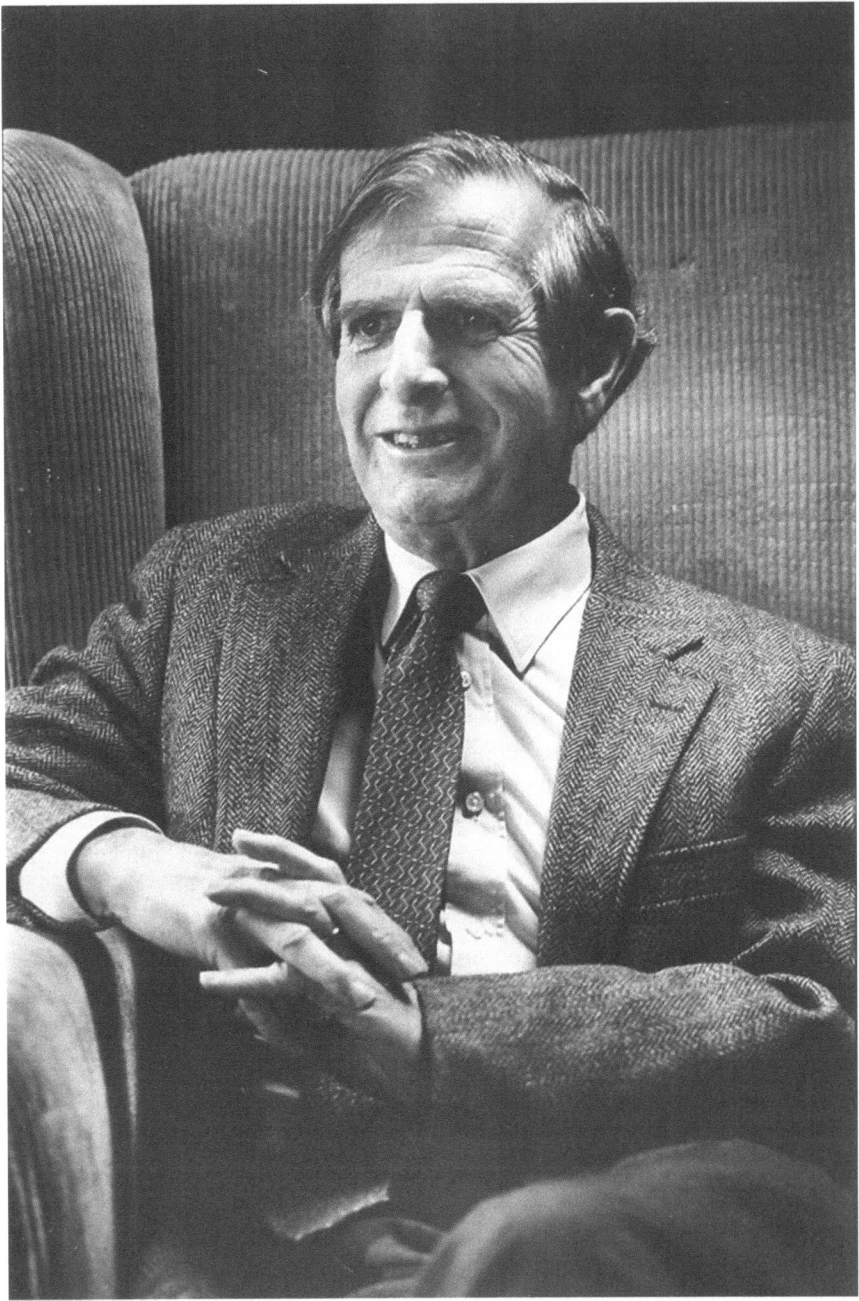

Fig. 10: Dr. Louis Micheels, 1989.
(courtesy of the Micheels' family)

3 Dr Gisella Perl

The Nazi method of completely dehumanizing us before throwing us into the fire worked beautifully. Only a very few, the strongest, the cleanest, the noblest were able to retain a semblance of human dignity; the rest were engulfed by the gurgling swamp of crime, mental deterioration and filth. (Gisella Per 1984, 37)

Gisella Perl was born on the 10 December 1892[32] in the town of Sighet[33] in Transylvania, at a time when it was part of Romania. Known as Giske, she lived with her parents, Moris (Moshe) and Phrida (Phridelle) and six brothers and sisters. Moris, a loving but strict father, was a successful businessman providing the family with all the comforts of life. Phrida was a loving, supportive wife and mother. The family was Orthodox Jewish. Perl's early life and adolescence centred on family, education and religious observance with Gisella and her brothers and sister studying the Torah four to five hours a day. Her value-system was grounded from the love of her parents the close relationship with her brothers and sisters and religious observance. She was bright at school attending Litzen high school in Sighet coming first in her final year. Apart from the recollections of her daughter, Ella, and grandson, Giora, little is known of Gisella's early life. With the exception of her sister Helen, and daughter Ella, all members of her family perished in Auschwitz. From early life Perl's ambition was to become a doctor, and despite her father's protests Perl and her sister Helen graduated in medicine. Her father

---

32 According to Gisella Perl's daughter Ella and grandson Giora (Kraus & Yardeni 2011) she was born in 1892. Later, Giora explained (in an email to the author) that Perl was known to fudge her age and that her passport stated she was born in 1892. Another source (Brozan 1982) contends she was born in 1900 or 1910. When the matter of her age is investigated, 1910 does not fit the timeline for Gisella would have been 12 when Imre was born and 18 when Ella was born. If she was born in 1900 Gisella would have married when she was about 20 years old yet it is reported that when she married, both her husband and Gisella were doctors.

33 Sighet, now Sighetu Marmatei, Romania, is located on the Tisza River in northern Transylvania. It is the birthplace of Elie Wiesel. From the late 18th century it was a centre of Orthodox and Chassidic Jewish life. The first Jewish families arrived in Sighet in approximately 1720. By 1740 there were sufficient Jews for a permanent Minyan and by 1787 the population of Jews represented about four per cent of the population of Sighet numbering 3495 residents. During the 19th century the Jewish community grew rapidly to represent approximately 39 per cent of the population by 1941. Sighet had the highest proportion of Jews of any town or city in Hungary most of whom were Orthodox. The period between 1860 and the First World War was a special time for the Jews and while refusing to assimilate completely into the general community, they played a prominent role in business, the professions and government. In Sighet, leading families including the Perl's, amassed considerable wealth from investment in commercial enterprises such as forestry and transport. The majority of the Jews in Sighet were Yiddish speaking and reluctant to assimilate.

https://doi.org/10.1515/9783110598216-006

argued that daughters should adhere to Jewish tradition, finding a successful husband, raising children and attending to wifely duties, particularly running a Kosher home. He was afraid they would be lost to their faith. However, Perl persisted, promising her father that she would never abandon her religion. After graduating, she bought her father a *Tanakh*,[34] and inscribed in it that she would always continue to embrace the Jewish religion and life. She contends her father took the Tanakh to Auschwitz and had it with him when he went into the gas chamber.[35] Taking anything into the gas chambers was impossible as the people were stripped naked after being told they were taking a shower. At the time Perl may have meant that her father took the bible to the gas chamber not knowing he could not take it into the death chamber.

According to Ella Kraus & Yardeni (2011), Gisella was a stubborn and determined child and adolescent who always got her way, a trait that she carried throughout her life. In 1920 Perl and Ephraim Kraus, a doctor, were married. They established a medical practice in Sighet, Gisella as a gynaecologist and her husband in general practice. On 31 December 1922 Imre (Emerik) was born and six years later on 25 August 1928, Ella[36] (Gabriella) was born. Life for Gisella and Ephraim and the family was happy and peaceful. The photo of the Perl/Kraus family as depicted in Fig. 11 shows a flourishing well presented family. Gisella and Ephraim were doctors and Ella and Imre were attending school. They enjoyed their success living in a beautiful house that had belonged to Cornelia Priel, the great Hungarian artist of French origin. Prior to the Great War, Jews in Sighet and

---

34 The *Tanakh* is a name used in Judaism for the canon of the Hebrew Bible. The *Tanakh* is also known as the *Miqra*. The name is an acronym formed from the initial Hebrew letters of the Masoretic Text's three traditional sub-divisions: *The Torah* ('Teaching' also known as the Five Books of Moses) *Nevi im* (Prophets) and *Ketuvim* ('Writing') – hence TaNaKh

35 Perl's father could not take it into the chambers unless he smuggled it somehow. He may have taken it to Auschwitz and it is highly likely it would have been taken from him immediately upon arrival. It is impossible to know what happened to the *Tanakh* and it must be assumed this is what Perl wanted to happen.

36 In the chapter the *Evaluation of Sources* the absence of Ella is discussed and the apparent distortion of the age and fate of Imre. In neither her memoirs nor a movie made of her life in Auschwitz and her arrival in the United States does Perl mention her daughter Ella. It is as if Ella never existed. In interviews with Ella and her son Giora neither could explain why Gisella failed to mention Ella. Imre is referred to in both the book and movie as the only child who travelled to the ghettos and Auschwitz. According to Ella her brother was twenty-two years of age in 1944 when he was sent to a labour camp and shot in his attempt to escape. In two postcards sent by Gisella and her mother to both Ella and Helen from the ghetto before shipment to Auschwitz mention is made of the relatives who were with them. Imre is not mentioned as being with the group going to Auschwitz and, in fact, Gisella asks Ella and Helen to look after Imre. The evidence reveals Imre was not with Perl in Auschwitz.

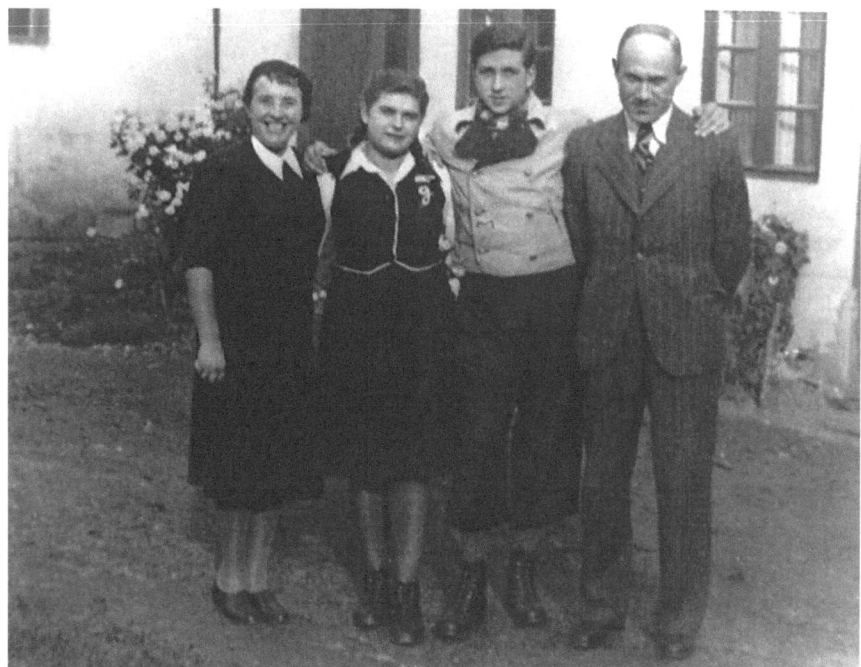

Fig. 11: Gisella Perl, Ella, (daughter) Imre (son), and Ephraim (husband).
(courtesy of Ella Kraus, daughter and Giora Kraus, grandson of Gisella Perl)

Hungary lived a relatively peaceful and uninterrupted life successful in most areas of business and the professions. Unlike the early life of Jews in many towns and cities throughout Europe, Perl did not suffer antisemitism at school or from the non-Jewish community.

The end of the Great War in 1918 witnessed gradual changes for the Jews in Hungary with growing resentment of disproportionate Jewish representation in the professions and business.[37] Resentment toward the Jews became widespread and Regent Miklos Horthy declared he was an antisemite, and remarked in a letter to his prime minister:

> I have considered it intolerable that here in Hungary everything, every factory, bank, large fortune, business, theatre, press, commerce, etc. should be in Jewish hands, and that the Jew should be the image reflected of Hungary, especially abroad. (Patai 1996, 546)

---

[37] In 1920, 60 per cent of Hungarian doctors, 51 per cent of lawyers, 39 per cent of all privately employed engineers and chemists, 34 per cent of editors

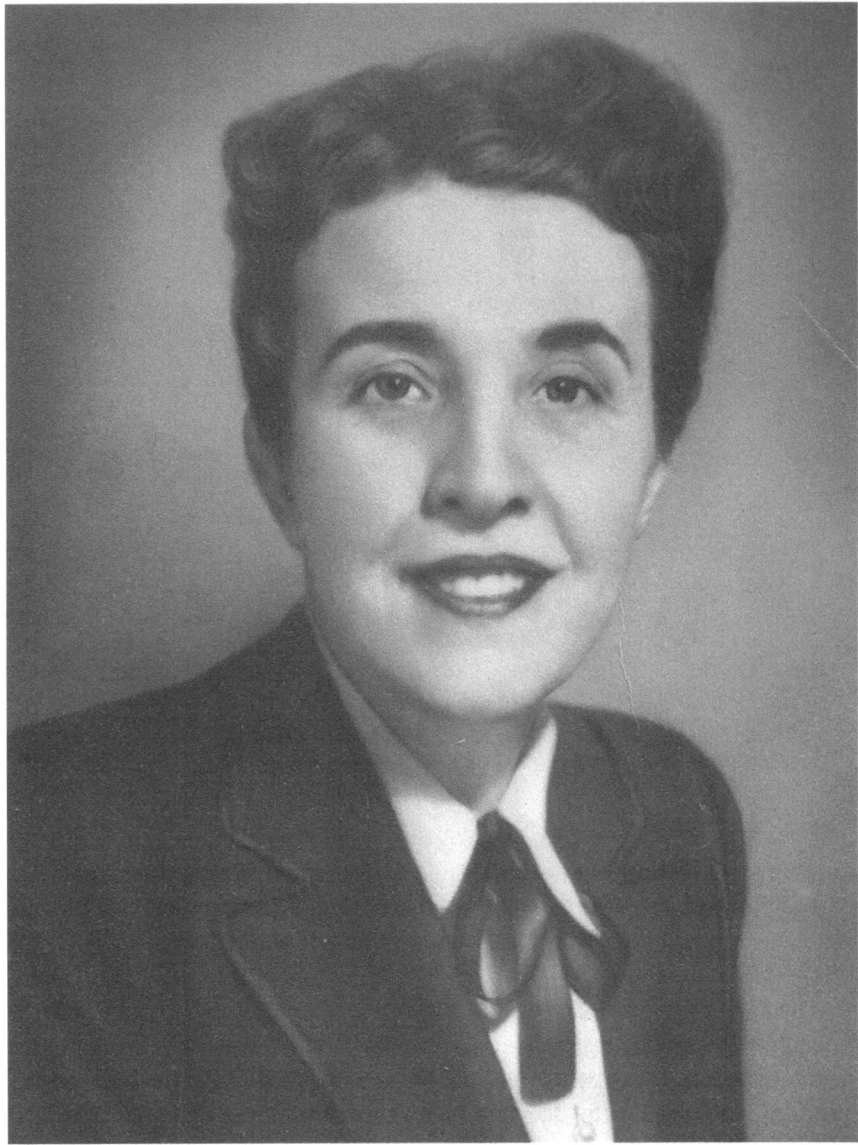

Fig. 12: Gisella as a young doctor before Auschwitz. (courtesy of Ella Kraus and Giora Kraus)

From 1920 until 1940 the Hungarian government introduced laws to reduce the power and influence of Jews in Hungarian life. By the late 1930s and early 1940s life for the Jews of Sighet became very difficult and initially there was pressure discouraging them from furthering their interests in business and the professions.

Pressure was transformed into legislation banning Jews from Hungarian life. By 1943 Perl feared for her family's safety:

> Within the walls of my green salon, surrounded by the love and admiration of my husband and son ... it was there that every evening I gathered the strength and will to continue my work that was becoming increasingly difficult. (Perl, 1984, 15)

By early 1944 the situation in Hungary became hopeless for the Jews. The Nazis were putting more and more pressure on the Hungarian government to take decisive action against the Jews. The frustration of the Nazis was not one-dimensional:

> There was a close correlation between the succession of Hungarian rulers and the pacing of the anti-Jewish action. The moderate prime ministers slowed down and arrested the catastrophe; the extremists hurried it along ... near tranquillity alternated with outbursts of destructive activity. (Hilberg 1985, 799)

In March 1944 Horthy succumbed to the pressure and threats and 'legitimized the (German) occupation and contributed to the placement of the entire Hungarian state apparatus at the service of the Germans.'[38] Despite the looming disaster for the Perl family, Gisella became pro-active trying to persuade her mother and father and family to escape from Hungary. Her actions showed the deep love for her family and her determination to try to save them from what she saw as the coming catastrophe. The severity and brutality of the times, the seizure of all assets including homes and businesses, the requirement to wear the Star of David, the humiliations and the level of indiscriminate violence forced Perl and her siblings to confront their parents again pleading with them to escape to a safer country. At this stage, they still had the means and contacts to leave for a safe haven. Despite the looming peril Moris and his wife refused to leave Sighet under any circumstance and demanded the family stay together. They were in denial as to the true motives of the Nazis, believing the Hungarian government

---

38 Miklós Horthy an Admiral of the Austro-Hungarian Navy was chosen as the Regent to represent the monarchy of Hungary after the Allies would not accept the return of Charles IV to the throne. This was despite a coalition of right-wing political forces on 1 March, 1920, uniting and returning Hungary to a Constitutional Monarchy. Sándor Simonyi-Semadam was the first Prime Minister of Horthy's Regency. Hungary went through a turbulent time from the 1920s until the end of the Second World War with several Prime Ministers all of whom had different agendas. Horthy wanted to appease both the wealthy who controlled the economy, mostly the Jews and the anti-Semites. Fearing a Soviet invasion Horthy deposed the last fascist Prime Minister and installed an anti-Fascist regime in an effort to appease the allies. However, the Nazis invaded Hungary, installed Ferenc Szálisa of the anti-Semitic and the pro-Nazi Arrow Cross Party to form a puppet government. From May to June 1944 approximately 500,000 Jews were sent to their death, most to Auschwitz.

would protect them.[39] At this time Perl and Ella were in Bucharest where Perl was working with her sister at a hospital. The parents demanded all family members return to Sighet, but Helen refused to return and Perl, while deciding to obey her parents, asked Helen to keep Ella with her in Bucharest. On 19 March 1944, the Nazis gained absolute power over Hungary and put into motion the destruction of the Jewish population. The Jewish community of Sighet was not spared the wrath of the Nazis as Perl recounts:

> Quickly, quickly, so as to squeeze their whole beastly program into a short time they began bombarding us with order after order. First we had to sew on the yellow Star of David ... then came the curfew ... travel was prohibited ... homes were searched ... people interned ... stores, business requisitioned ... endless succession of sudden alarms. Then came an order forbidding us to leave our houses for three days ... Police broke into house after house, demanding gold, silver, jewels, valuables and money. They ... took everything they fancied, unmindful of our presence as though we were already dead. (Perl, 1984, 17)

In the case of Perl's immediate and extended family all material possessions were lost and their social status and professional reputation destroyed. Their beautiful homes and lifestyle were replaced by ghetto existence. The family, so successful and united, was thrown into a foreign world of humiliation and despair. The parents' refusal to escape had devastating consequences with only Perl and her daughter and sister surviving. Imre was sent to a labour camp while Ella and Helen were in Bucharest with a plan to escape the Nazi terror (Kraus & Yardeni 2011). Both were fortunate in finding sanctuary with two Christian families. Ella stayed with the Chashar family who believed she was a Christian Hungarian girl[40] Ella was a young blonde girl who did not have the distinctive features of a Jewess (Kraus & Yardeni 2011). Gisella and her mother, Phrida, sent the following postcards[41] to Ella:

---

39 In regard to Sighet and the fate of the Jews, François Mauriac writes: 'Their blindness as they confronted a destiny from which they would have still had time to flee; the inconceivable passivity with which they surrendered to it, deaf to the warnings and pleas of a witness (Moishe the Beadle) who escaped a massacre and recounts his experiences which the Jews of Sighet refuse to believe' (Wiesel 2006, xviii).

40 According to Ella when Helen came to take her at the end of the war the Chashar family wanted to adopt her and bring her up as their own child (Kraus & Yardeni 2011).

41 There were two types of post cards. When Jews arrived in the camps the Nazis would supply a post card that provided the recipient with a glowing picture of life in the camp, the wonderful life of plentiful food and accommodation, medical care and constant work in the fields. This strategy was aimed at encouraging the Jews to join the members of the family and friends at the camps. Once the truth became known the post cards became ineffective. Sending this postcard to Ella and Imre was apparently allowed in this particular ghetto.

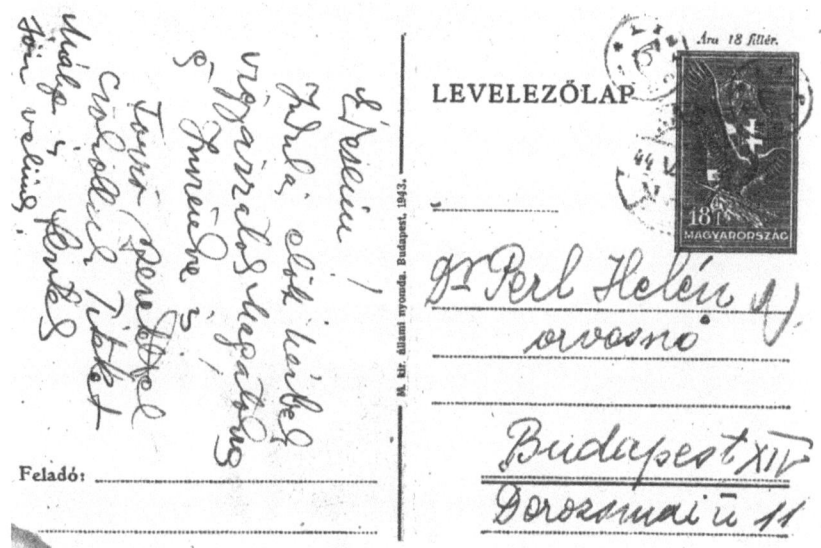

Fig. 13: Post card from the grandmother to Ella (grand daughter).(Courtesy of Ella Kraus and Giora Kraus Daughter and Grandson of Gisella)

Dear Ella!

Please take care of each other [Ella and her aunt Helen] and also Imre. Mia is also going with us

Loving you, kisses, full of love.

Granny

and:

Dear children!

We are at Solomon Street, in the schoolyard. Together with us are Granddaddy and Granny, [Dr Perl's parents], uncle Bella and his wife [Dr Perl's brother], Doodi and his sick wife, father Pherike [Dr Perl's husband Ephraim] and myself.

We are leaving now, and when we will arrive at the end and if possible, we will write you. We are praying, begging and hoping that it will be possible to write to you again.

All my life I loved and take care of you, now you need to take care and love each other. Loving you with all my heart, we are leaving now.

Giske

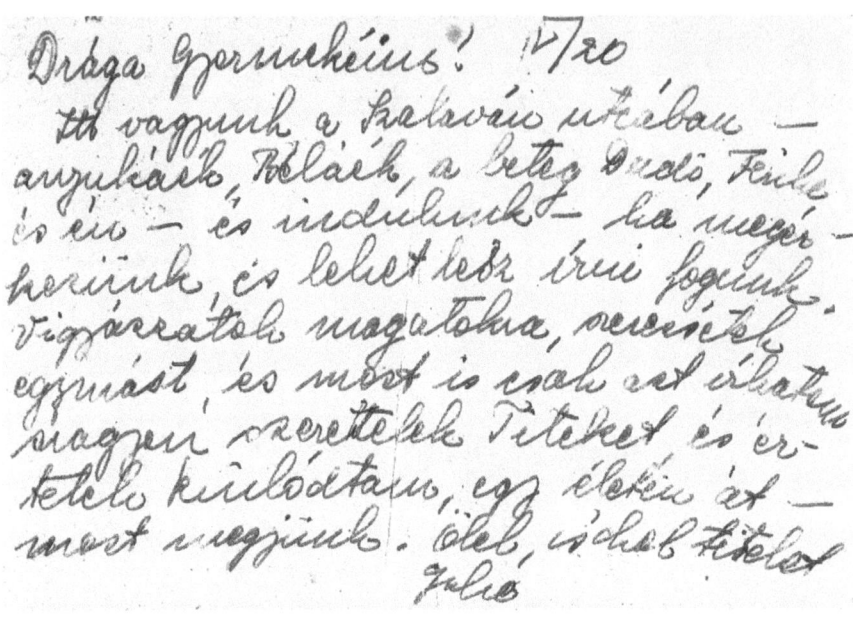

Fig. 14: Postcard Post card from Gisella writing from the ghetto to her children Imre and Ella. (Courtesy of Ella Kraus and Giora Kraus Daughter and Grandson of Gisella)

The postcard from Prida to Ella is very important for it confirms that first she existed, second she was a family member and finally she did not go to Auschwitz with the family. Perl addressed her card to her *'children'* and named the members of the family in the ghetto. Imre is not mentioned.[42] The postcard conveyed a sense of despair and foreshadowed the fear that it could be the last contact made with her children. The period in the ghetto, although of relatively short duration, was the harbinger of their fate. Perl described the living conditions with eight to ten persons sharing a room in dilapidated shacks, a far cry from the beautiful family home once owned by Priel. Despite the terrible conditions Perl did not fall into despair and saw hope in hopelessness:

> We could still watch the sun go down over our mountains and we could still hope in our hearts that our liberators would soon come down the mountain slopes. We had our friends and our relatives around us, and their love brightened the fear that filled our souls. (Perl 1984, 18)

---

42 This point is important because in her memoirs Gisella does not mention her daughter yet she devotes a chapter to Elizabeth, a young gentile whom she takes into her home. Gisella recalls Elizabeth and Imre sharing a close relationship. Ella is not mentioned.

However, despair and humiliation came with the intrusive behaviour of the Gestapo men when examining the women[43] for hidden valuables 'I had to stand by and watch while they seized one woman after another and with dirty fingers searched the depths of her body for treasures' (Perl 1984, 26). Hope came when Perl was directed to establish a hospital and a maternity ward in the ghetto. Fully convinced this directive could only mean that the ghetto was going to be a permanent home until the end of the war, Gisella enthusiastically launched into her assignment only to discover that once established, a counter-directive came for immediate deportation of all Jews. For Gisella and her family, the destination was Auschwitz. This was Gisella's first experience of the Nazis' strategy in breaking the Jewish people in both body and mind. It was also a control issue, the Nazis demonstrating they had absolute power over the Jews. Perl's recognition of the contradictory behaviour of her tormentors and their mind games was to her advantage. She became aware of the mechanism of control and came to understand their methods.

The next stage began with the infamous train trip to Auschwitz. Gisella recalls the trip of eight days, day and night, crammed into cattle cars with the doors sealed and only a sliver of light and air. The cars held eighty to one hundred people who for most of the trip went without food or water.

> The small children cried with hunger and cold, the old people moaned for help, some went insane, others gave life to their babies there on the dirty floor, some died and their bodies travelled with us ... Once in a while our jailers would enter the car in a renewed search for valuables, or only to silence plaintive voices with brutal threats. (Perl 1984, 30)

Did this experience affect her confidence and test her resilience and determination? Although she had witnessed inhumanity in the ghetto, the train trip was another experience altogether encompassing a level of suffering she could not have imagined. This becomes apparent when she attempts suicide soon after arrival in the camp. The train trip and her treatment upon entering the camp spiralled her into a state of despair. At the ramp an SS doctor, possibly Josef Mengele, directed prisoners to the right or left. With the exception of Perl, her family was sent to the left and to their death. She said goodbye to her father, mother and brothers and sisters, as her entire family were loaded into Red Cross trucks, in a weird mockery of all human decency, and carted away; and all we ever saw of them again were their clothes in the storeroom of the camp (Perl 1984, 28). From the ramp Perl walked to

---

43 Judaism states that clothing the body adds dignity to the person and women are encouraged to be modest in appearance. Respect for a women and her body is paramount to the purity of family life. The actions of the Nazis, were a gross violation of the Jewish women, but were in line with the process of dehumanization of the individual.

the camp, and during the march she was to witness what was to become a common sight, rotting corpses. At the camp, they commenced the initiation process. The Nazis were met with violent resistance from the terrified prisoners.

> But suddenly the column disintegrated, the unbearable tension exploded and the terror, the pain, the sorrow, and the loneliness turned women into screaming, panicky, and hysterical creatures. They refused to enter the building that had the sign Disinfection painted on it in large letters. Bullets flew, whips cracked and clubs fell with a dull sound, leaving broken bones and open skulls in their wake. (Perl 1984, 29)

The prisoners were in a state of despair and fear before they arrived at the camp compounds. The sight of dead bodies, likely in a state of decay, the smell of burnt flesh and the general conditions of filth they witnessed knowing this was to be their home aroused unimaginable anxiety and terror. By 1944 there was no doubt the newly arrived prisoners knew their fate and thus fear and hysteria were not an uncommon reaction. As a doctor, Perl was commanded under the threat of death to quiet the hysterical women. She successfully did by promising they would be safe. Yet they were executed. She did not know what was to happen to the prisoners but acted to save her own life. During the initiation period the prisoners were shaved of every hair on their bodies. They entered the special rooms at least human like:

> Above all, we still had our identity, our individuality that made us different from other women around us, and our pride, which, as we learned, gets most of its support from outer appearances. (Perl 1984, 43)

Perl and the other female prisoners left the room leaving behind their only remaining possessions, their identity, appearance, dignity and name that was replaced by number. As Perl recalls 'Our heads had acquired a nightmarish appearance, cropped close by unskilled hands, so horrible to look at that we did not know whether to laugh or to cry' (Perl 1984, 44). It was at this point she attempted suicide. She was overwhelmed by the cruelty and depravity and lost hope:

> When we came out of the building we did not know each other anymore. Instead of the exhausted, tortured, but still self-respecting women who entered through its door, we were a heart-rending lot of crying clowns, a ghastly carnival procession marching toward the last festival: death. (Perl 1984, 32)

Her storage of optimism, resilience and determination had evaporated. Her first impression of camp life began with the sight of a never-ending row of dark, filthy, rat-infested wooden blocks. To her horror each block equipped to house four hundred held approximately twelve hundred prisoners.

Along the inner walls of the barracks, there were three rows of wooden shelves, one above the other, and these shelves were our bedrooms, living rooms, dining rooms and studies, all in one. They were divided by vertical planks at regular intervals. Each of these cage-like contraptions served as sleeping-room for thirty to thirty-six persons. Once in a while the shelves would collapse under the weight of the sleepers and the inmates fell on one another in a bloody medley of broken bones, bleeding wounds, loud wailing, and, more often than not, a whipping by the Blockova or block superintendent. (Perl 1984, 33)

However, the sanitary conditions were the most shocking to Perl where excrement was everywhere to the extent they were often knee-deep in human waste. Des Pres created the term 'excremental assault' to describe the conditions and explain the level of debasement to which the prisoners were subject. Everyone suffered from diarrheal or dysentery and in camps such as Birkenau that were awash with excreta, prisoners walked in the waste of patients who suffered from highly contagious diseases.

Those with dysentery melted down like candles, relieving themselves in their clothes, and swiftly turned into stinking repulsive skeletons who died in their own excrement. (Donat 1958, 269)

The conditions were used as a tool to break the morality, dignity and self-worth of the prisoner, as Des Pres described:

Prisoners were systematically subjected to filth ... Defilement was a constant threat, a condition of life from day to day, and at any moment it was liable to take abruptly vicious and sometimes fatal forms. (Des Pres 1976, 57)

Des Pres contends that SS actions and behaviour were not random but were a deliberate policy of destroying the prisoner physically, mentally and emotionally. The SS guards had the power to kill anyone they saw fit, however, merely killing was not enough. Absolute power was the goal of the Nazis, to first completely break the soul of the Jewish prisoner and then kill him or her.

The pathological rage of such men, their uncontrollable fury when rules were broken, is evidence of the boundless desire to annihilate, to destroy, to smash everything not mobilized within the movement of their own authority. And inevitably, the mere act of killing is not enough; for if a man dies without surrender, if something within him remains unbroken to the end, then the power that destroyed him has not, after all, crushed everything. (Des Pres 1976, 57)

In the initial stage of camp life Perl was not assigned to a hospital or infirmary, but to labour work. Despite her situation she initiated caring for the prisoners in her block. Food and water were scarce. Each prisoner could take ten sips of the watery soup. Sometimes when the containers were taken to blocks, the prisoners who had already had their portions would attack the carriers. Violent fighting would break out and according to Gisella her busiest period was after dinner from the fighting:

> There were bleeding heads to bandage, broken ribs to be taped, scratches to be cleaned, burn wounds to be soothed. I worked and worked, knowing only too well that it was hopeless, because tomorrow everything would begin again, even the patients would be the same. (Perl 1984, 41)

At such an early stage in the camp helping prisoners would have enhanced her self-esteem and confidence. Even under such conditions she could still help others. Unlike some Jewish doctors who were assigned to research institutes or special blocks, Perl worked in Birkenau in the women's camp where conditions were atrocious. Perl as a prisoner doctor was considered a 'privileged' prisoner but in name only. She lived in the worst conditions:

> We sank deeper and deeper into sub-human existence where filth, pain, and crime were natural, and a decent impulse, a human gesture something to be sneered at and disbelieved ... for two months I had stood on my bare feet during the two daily roll calls. I had no shoes. My feet swelled up and were covered with sores – which was not only painful but also dangerous. (Perl 1984, 56)

Footwear was a precious item in the camp. For a prisoner with ill-fitting shoes, the feet would develop blisters that became worse as time passed which would prevent him or her from working. This usually meant death. The lack of footwear altogether was a potential death sentence as well. In an effort to secure shoes and laces Perl experienced an event that was so disgusting and reprehensible that from her state of despair and angst arose a determination not to let the culture of cruelty and putrefaction defeat her. 'I could not permit myself to be engulfed in this swamp of human depravity (Perl 1984, 65). Des Pres maintains that,

> ... by choosing not only to live, but to live humanly, they (the survivors) take upon themselves the burden of action requiring much will and courage, much clear-sightedness and faith in life. (Des Pres 1976, 57)

A profound change in Perl occurred when she was sold a pair of shoes. A fellow prisoner stole a pair of shoes from the crematorium. The price was two-days of bread rations, a price Perl eagerly paid. Unfortunately, the shoes did not have laces. That made walking difficult, causing blisters. Told that she could get string in exchange for food in the latrine, Perl went to the latrine[44] where most bartering was done. To her horror this male prisoner did not want bread, but sex.

---

44 The latrine was an important part of the camp for it was where a prisoner could barter.

[He was] a short, stocky, pockmarked man with wild eyes and a ferocious expression. The inferno Auschwitz had succeeded in depriving him of his last vestige of human dignity ... for a second I didn't understand what he meant. I asked him again, smiling, gently, to give me a piece of string ... My feet were killing me ... The shoes were useless without string ... It might save my life ... he wasn't listening to me. 'Hurry up ... hurry up ...' he said hoarsely. His hand, filthy with excrement he was working in, reached out for my womanhood, rudely, insistently. (Perl 1984, 58)

The experience became a manifestation of rage and revenge. It was not only her personal degradation but the realization of the level to which she had sunk, and Perl was not going to allow her dignity to be taken away from her. 'Yes, I was going to remain a human being to the last minute of my life – whenever that would come' (Perl 1984, 59). Another experience made her resolve even stronger and set her on a path that shaped her purpose and gave her life meaning while in the camp. During roll call, Mengele, in an effort to identify pregnant women, ordered Perl to tell the women that they could give birth, and both mother and baby would receive proper care.

He had them put into a special, so-called 'obstetric block,' where they actually got double rations. Many deluded women believed that they would be allowed to give birth in peace ... his interest was so great that he would be present at every birth, but immediately afterwards the infants were sent to the gas chamber. I can testify to this as it was my duty to examine and report to him all the pregnant women. I was even forced to bring the infants to the gas chamber ... one night he rushed like a devil into the 'obstetric' block stabbing the mothers in the abdomen, shooting about with his revolver, singing, laughing in demonic mirth. Then the whole block was burnt. One of the mothers was in the middle of birth pains with the infant's head appearing. Mengele, like fury, dragged her by the feet, and with his own hands put her into the death car (Perl, 1947)[45]

The two experiences produced a fundamental and lasting change in Perl both personally and professionally. In the case of the former she resolved not to give up but to survive and professionally she was committed to save as many pregnant women as humanly possible. Witnessing pregnant women beaten and thrown into death wagons and then into the ovens alive touched a nerve that led to an obsession.

I stood, rooted to the ground, unable to move, to scream, to run away. But gradually the horror turned into revolt and this revolt shook me out of my lethargy and gave me a new incentive to live. I had to remain alive. It was up to me to save all the pregnant women in

---

45 Letter by Gisella Perl sent to the Office of the US Chief of Counsel, War Department, Washington, DC, 11 January 1947, offering herself as a witness at a trial of Mengele. Perl mistakenly believed Mengele had been captured and was to stand trial.

> Camp C from this infernal fate. It was up to me to save the life of the mothers, if there was no
> other way, than by destroying the life of their unborn children. (Perl 1984, 81)

Perl's traits combined with her experiences of her past life gradually took shape. From an early age she was stubborn and resolute. Her determination to become a doctor was uncompromising and single-minded. She became determined and self-assured. She showed resilience by rising from the depths of despair and embraced a cause that gave meaning to her life. She showed concern and sympathy for all patients but particularly pregnant women. Perl instructed all pregnant women to hide their condition from anyone in authority even the Blockova (prisoner in charge of a block). It was essential for her to know when a woman fell pregnant to enable her to abort the child:

> On dark nights, when everyone else was sleeping – in dark corners of the camp, in the toilet,
> on the floor, without a drop of water, I delivered their babies. First I took the nine-month
> pregnancies, I accelerated the birth by the rupture of the membranes, and usually within
> one or two days spontaneous birth took place without intervention. Or I produced dilation
> with my fingers, inverted the embryo and thus brought it to life. (Perl 1984, 81)

Perl delivered babies when the women were at all stages of pregnancy in the most inhuman conditions. Initially she was overwhelmed with grief and guilt but knew that by aborting the child or killing the newborn baby she was saving the life of the mother. Officially Gisella worked in Block 19 with four Jewish doctors and four nurses. They formed a tight supportive group and worked hard to keep their sanity and self-respect. Some doctors, including Perl, were fortunate enough to have the opportunity to treat 'private' patients, those who needed treatment and could afford to pay with either food or valuables. With the proceeds, Perl would barter urgently needed medical supplies and medicines.

Gisella's life in Auschwitz was a landscape littered with inhumanity. According to Perl she didn't experience the so-called luxuries of some other Jewish doctors such as better clothing and shoes, more comfortable and clean-living conditions and better medical equipment or supplies. Birkenau was a death camp with a brief to kill all prisoners. Why would the Nazis spend time and energy in providing better conditions and facilities? Unlike some Jewish doctors, Gisella did not live in a cocoon shielded from some of the worst cases of brutality and bestiality.

> As I watched, I saw two beautiful eyes disappear under a layer of blood ... Her ears weren't
> there any longer, maybe he had torn them off ... And in a few seconds her straight pointed
> nose was a flat, broken, bleeding mass. I closed my eyes, unable to bear it any longer, and
> when I opened them again Dr Mengele had stopped hitting her. But instead of a human
> head, Ibis's tall, thin body carried a round, blood red object on its bony shoulders, an

unrecognizable object, too horrible to look at. As he pushed her back into line and her long emaciated legs took on the rhythm of the march, the bleeding head before my eyes turned into a globe, and it seemed to me as if Ibis's victimized body were [sic] carrying our worn-torn, doomed Earth into the flames .... (Perl 1984, 111)

How did Perl survive this inhumanity? How did she not go insane? In an interview with me in Sydney, Alex Lowy (2011), a survivor of Mauthausen concentration camp, recalled an experience on the Death march when a fellow prisoner, his friend, could not continue and stopped and sat down to rest. A guard approached him and kicked the young boy to death. The boy's father jumped on the boy's body to protect his son, whereupon another guard shot the father in the head. I asked Mr Lowy what his reaction to such brutality was. At that point he became emotional and explained to me that death and savagery had replaced life and to survive he was forced to rise above the pain and horror and disconnect from the realities of the life of which they had become immersed. He had witnessed so much violence, depravity and death it did not affect him and he could not let it do so. He would have gone insane. Yet during our meeting Mr Lowy became upset revealing how dramatically the experience of living through the Holocaust had impacted his life. Did Perl become immune? Was this the only way she could continue to abort babies and kill newborn babies?

Perl's trip to her next camp was fortuitous for she did not go on the same journey as those on the infamous Death March. She was ordered by Mengele to accompany two SS guards:

I was walking over the snow and ice of the outskirts of the camp in my men's shoes of yellow leather, between two cruelly silent SS guards, into uncertainty, maybe into death ... the barbed wire fence disappeared in the fog between us. The crematory did not function any longer and the sky was as grey and merciless as the ground under my feet. (Perl 1984, 142)

Perl and her guards walked throughout the day and night until they came to Katowice, a large city that she remembered first passing on her way to Auschwitz. Arriving in Berlin by train she continued her journey to a concentration camp outside Hamburg. She was assigned to the Arbeitslager, a labour camp, situated in the suburb of Wandsbek. The hospital was at Dege-Werke, a rubber plant serving the Nazi war effort. Shortly after her arrival Perl was told she would be in charge of the hospital. Once again she was under the threat of punishment and death:

If you try to run away you'll be caught and hanged ... and remember, I don't want too many patients in that hospital of yours ... I make you responsible for them and you'll be beaten if I find any malingerers in bed. (Perl 1984, 154)

Perl was again in the same hospital environment as she had been in Auschwitz. She discovered Auschwitz had been liberated and she said she 'went around in a red haze of pain, despair, fury (Perl 1984, 155). Obviously, she was not aware of the true picture of the fate of her fellow prisoners, all of whom went on the Death March that claimed thousands of lives. Perl's rage subsided and she continued to devote her energies to caring for sick and beaten Jews. The allied bombing did not spare the labour and concentration camps, and Perl and her colleagues were required to attend an increasing number of victims:

> The wounded were brought in incessantly, with arms and legs torn off by bombs, deep wounds in the heads, their ribs crushed by falling bricks, some more dead than alive. All day long I sewed, bandaged, put broken limbs in plaster and gave a few moments of respite from pain to the dying ... my ears were filled with the shrieking of the sirens and the moans of the bomb victims. (Perl 1984, 159)

Although she knew the war would soon end, she was sent to Bergen Belsen, referred to as a 'dung-heap' by the Nazis. Perl described her situation:

> It was supreme fulfilment of German sadism and bestiality ... can never be described because every language lacks the suitable words to depict its horrors. It cannot be imagined, because even the most pathological mind balks at such a picture. One must have seen those mountains of rotting corpses mixed with filth, with human excrement, where once in a while one noticed a slight movement caused by rats or by the death convulsion of a victim who had been thrown there alive. One must have smelled the unimaginable stench that lay over the camp like a thick cloud shutting out the air. One must have heard those unearthly screams of agony that continued through the day and the night, coming from hundreds of throats, unceasingly, unbearably. (Perl 1984, 167)

Did this camp finally exhaust all of Perl's energy? Obviously in Auschwitz she could not have imagined that anything could be worse. The new camp may have been the final test of her resilience and hardiness. But it did not deter her from caring for and helping those suffering and close to death. Perl received a commemoration from the British commander of Bergen Belsen for her services to camp patients. Tragically it was during this period Perl discovered that her husband had been beaten to death and she claims her son had been cremated. The news appears to have finally broken her spirit and she attempted suicide only to be saved by a priest, Father Abbé Brand. After she recovered and through the efforts of Father Brand she applied for a 'priority certificate' through the Joint Distribution Committee and the Palestine Bureau to leave Europe. This was granted. In 1946 Perl arrived in New York under a temporary visa to participate in a series of lectures (sponsored by the Hungarian-Jewish Appeal and the United Jewish Appeal) explaining the horror of Jewish life under Nazism and raise funds for Jewish refugees. During these lectures two events took place that were to help her in her new life. Mrs Eleanor Roosevelt the wife of the former President of the United States of America attended one of her lectures and they became friends. They corresponded and Mrs Roosevelt, after becoming aware of Perl's history, encouraged her to resume her work as a gynaecologist, and she applied to gain permanent US residency. New York Representative Democrat Sol Bloom, petitioned the government to pass the bill that granted Perl her US visa. After a thorough investigation by the Justice Department of Perl's activities during her incarceration in Auschwitz and Bergen Belsen, President Harry Truman in 1948, signed a bill granting Perl residency in the US. Thereupon she retrained and qualified as a doctor in her new country. Perl commenced work in a New York hospital as a gynaecologist, and through the generosity of a friend lived in a fashionable part of New York City.

The second highlight of her life was finding her daughter alive and living in Israel. During a lecture she spoke of her daughter and mentioned her name and life before the war. A member of the audience recognized the name and told Perl he believed her daughter was living on a Kibbutz. Contact was made with Ella. In 1979 Perl moved to Israel and lived with her daughter. In Israel she volunteered her services as a gynaecologist at the *Shaare Zedek's gynaecology clinic* she delivered babies and helped those in need.

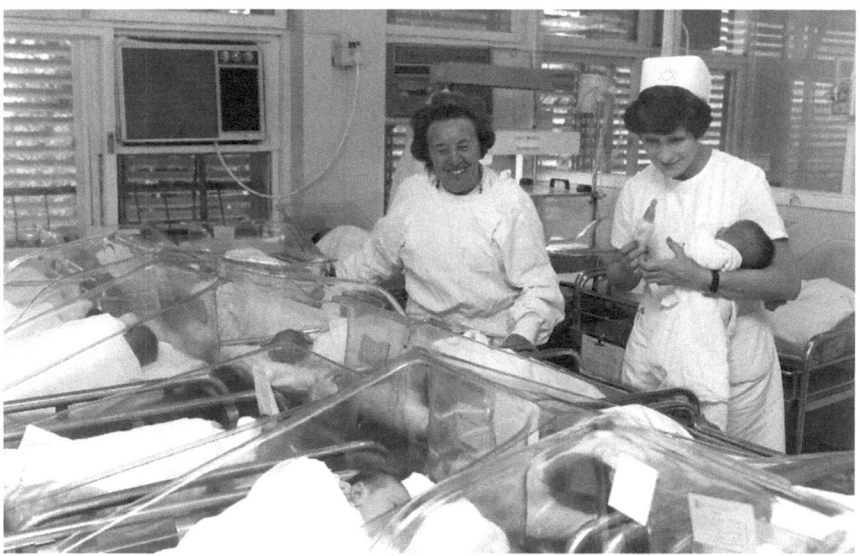

Fig. 15: Dr Gisella Perl in the gynaecology clinic of Shaare Zedek Medical Centre, Jerusalem. (courtesy of Ella Kraus and Giora Kraus)

Gisella Perl commenced life as a privileged individual and one would imagine she expected a successful and fulfilling life as a wife, mother and doctor. This life did not unfold for her. With the exception of her daughter and sister, her family perished. She experienced a world of inhumanity and evil that was impossible to comprehend. Her dedication to saving the lives of pregnant women was both courageous and altruistic but at a terrible price and was in most cases a paradox. She performed abortions and killed new-born babies to save pregnant women most of whom would die from the inhumane conditions of the camp. Despite the pain and suffering she endured during the Holocaust and guilt she felt after she survived to contribute to the betterment to humanity. Dr Gisella Perl passed away on Friday 16 December 1988 in Jerusalem.

In passing it is important to recognise Ella Straus was a Holocaust survivor. Ella lived with a protestant family who were not ware of her Jewish roots but she told me she was aware that they would have no hesitation to hand her to the SS if they became aware of her true identity. Her story of survival cannot be told here but it should be told at some time in the future.

Part III: **Jewish Physicians and the Hospital System**

Camp hospitals evoked fear in prisoners. As long as they could summon enough strength to stand, prisoners avoided sick call, which might place them in the hospital... Jews continued to be identified in hospitals as unfit for work and dispatched to the gas chambers
Yisrael Gutman (Gutman & Berenbaum 1998, 26)

The hospitals and infirmaries were another paradox. On the one hand they were places where prisoners, ill and injured, were kept alive to enable them to return to work. On the other hand, they were places where prisoners, as patients, were selected to die. The Jewish doctors were an integral part of this machinery. They were healers yet they took part in selections in which they were forced to make decisions condemning them to death.

After describing the hospital structure and conditions, I will describe the workings of the infamous Block 10, profiling two Jewish doctors, Alina Brewda and Maximilian Samuel, followed by examining the role of the Jewish doctor Lucie Adelsberger. We address the decisions made and actions taken by the doctors. Were they based on ethical dilemmas, choiceless choices or simply on the human condition? Under conditions of extreme adversity why do we expect a doctor to sacrifice his or her life for a person who faces imminent death? Primo Levi's concept of the Grey Zone is examined and applied to where the Jewish doctor stands within this zone. Among other important issues I examine the relationships between the Jewish doctors and the SS doctors and other non-Jewish, particularly Polish, prisoner doctors. The question of killing on the part of the Jewish doctors is discussed. Is there a difference between one type and another?

The issue of Jewish doctors working in the death comps is complicated and complex made so when they entered into the Nazi hospital system. Tragically they unwillingly but physically and actively became a part of an intentional and well-planned attempt to murder through a health system where safety and security is normally assured. By including Jewish and non-Jewish doctors in the process of suffering and death of prisoners in the name of medicine the actions of the Nazi doctors, to them, were legitimized. This is what makes the story and survival of some Jewish doctors interesting yet complex.

https://doi.org/10.1515/9783110598216-007

4 Hospitals and Infirmaries

I was trembling with excitement, with hope…Everything will be better now – I thought – we have a hospital for our sick, where they will be cured instead of being sent to the crematory. I'll be a doctor again, a healer, a reliever of human suffering. (Perl 1984, 70)

Little did Perl know these hopes would be shattered in a way that would change her life, exposing her to a side of humanity that was beyond her comprehension or her imagination. Over 350,000 Jews who entered the labour camps at Auschwitz were murdered either directly by execution or indirectly from exhaustion, starvation, disease and despair. Of those who were executed directly, tens of thousands were selected from the hospitals and infirmaries to be killed in the gas chambers or by phenol injection.

In 1940 when the camp was established, the camp medical centre, known as Abteilung V, was included in the organizational structure of the camp commandant's office.

In essence, there were two medical tiers: the official one, controlled by the SS, and the one of self-government by the prisoners. The official system was in keeping with the methodical, obsessive and brutal nature of Nazi officialdom. Until March 1942, Department V was directed by SS-Standartenführer Enno Lolling the chief SS garrison physician, who in turn coordinated the operations of three divisions: general medical, dental and pharmacological. Each of these divisions was in turn divided into a unit for the SS and a unit for the prisoners (Lasik et al. 2000). The SS Standortarzt was thus responsible for the state of health of the garrison, including both the SS personnel and the prison population and for all sanitary and hygienic installations. The camp physician, Lagerarzt, answered directly to the Standortarzt and to the chief physician of the SS SS-Obergruppenführer Ernst Robert von Grawitz[46] (Leitender Arzt der SS). Each received a monthly report detailing the medical situation in the camp as well as rates of sickness, infectious diseases and epidemics and the mortality for both the SS garrison and the prison population. These reports were also sent to the camp registry office, and the state and church administration offices (Lasik et al. 1995, 248).

---

46 Von Grawitz was a German physician and SS functionary. He was head of the German Red Cross and funded Nazi attempts to 'eradicate the perverted world of the homosexual' and research into attempts to 'cure' homosexuality (Lasik et al. 2000, 248).

https://doi.org/10.1515/9783110598216-008

Table 1: Organizational structure of department V in Auschwitz 1940–1945 (Lasik et al. 2000)

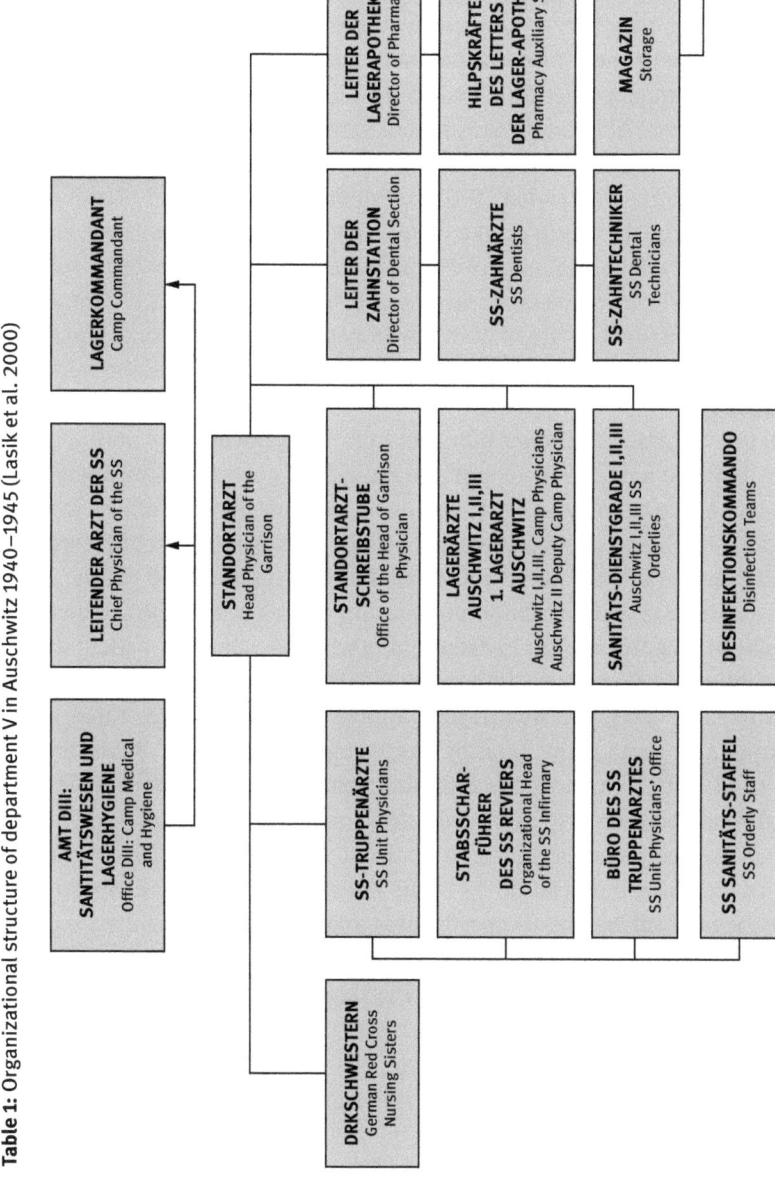

As the prison population increased from 700 in June 1940[47] to over 150,000 during various periods between 1942 and 1943, the hospital system expanded and changed. In March 1942 the medical service for concentration camps (Medizinischer Dienst der KL) was separated from the sanitary and hygiene division, and a new sanitary office division was established (Amt DIII – Sanitätswesen und Lagerhygiene). The head physician of concentration camps (Leitender Arzt) with the function of Head Office III became the executive physician and superior to the Standortarzt (Smoleń 1976, 8). Subordinate to the SS Standortarzt were: physicians of the SS detachments (SS Truppenärzte), responsible for the medical care of the SS personnel, SS camp physicians (SS Lagerärzte), responsible for the medical care of the camp prisoners, SS dental surgeons (SS Zahnärzte) responsible for the dental care of both the SS personnel and prisoners, and the SS apothecary (SS Lagerapotheker), who were in charge of the camp pharmacy (Czech 1990, 9).

With the increase in prisoner numbers from 1942, the hospital and infirmaries were assigned a dual role: to treat the injuries or illnesses of prisoners who would then be able to return to work, and to kill those who were too ill or weak to recover quickly. These prisoners were executed by phenol injection or gassed but their deaths were documented to appear as the result of illness so that no links could be made to an extermination program. In almost every case the hospital system played a significant role in determining whether a prisoner patient would live or die immediately or live a little longer to be worked to death.

In November 1943, the Auschwitz complex was divided into three separate camps: Auschwitz I, the main or base camp, Auschwitz II -Birkenau and Auschwitz III, which comprised mainly the labour camps and from November 1944 was renamed Monowitz. However, the change in camp structure did not result in a change of management or chain of command. The base camp KL Auschwitz remained the head office of the entire complex. The SS doctor had overall control of the health of the prisoners and SS staff and families, but the hospitals and infirmaries were largely administered by the political prisoners and criminals. The Lagerältester im Häftlingskrankenbau[48] was given primary

---

47 On May 20, 1940 the first prisoners consisting of 30 German criminals arrived and were appointed as prisoner functionaries. On June 14,1940 the first contingent of Polish prisoners, comprising 728 men, were sent to Auschwitz from Tarnów prison (Czech 1990, 13).
48 The *Häftlingskrankenbau* was the prisoner hospital. The *Lagerältester (the prisoner camp eldest)* wore a black armband inscribed 'LÄ'. He/she was senior to all prisoners except the *Krankenbauältester* (infirmary or hospital elder). *Blockältester* (block eldest): wore a red armband with a white label giving his function and block number; he/she was responsible for the administration of the block. The Stubendienste (prisoners on barracks-room duty) had to deal with food, clothing and cleanliness, and carried the food from the kitchen in pots.

authority to carry out the SS orders. Although medically unqualified, this was a prisoner the SS trusted to implement their policy and discipline. Reporting to the Lagerältester was the block senior – Blockältester – who was senior to and supervised the prisoner doctors. These supervisors were cruel and aggressive and at times as brutal as the SS. They assisted SS and prisoner doctors in selections and administration of phenol injections. It was not unusual for the Blockältester to operate on fellow prisoners despite a total lack of medical qualifications. Josef Klehr, a semi-literate Polish prisoner who had been a labourer before the war, earned the reputation as one of the most brutal functionaries in the camp. He murdered thousands of Jews by phenol injections. Lifton maintains that Klehr brought to Auschwitz enormous psychopathic potential, which the environment readily evoked. He argues that every society has a pool of Klehrs to draw upon for its killing assignments, and the medicalised dimension gave particular form to its extreme combination of sense of omnipotence, paranoid sadism, and schizoid numbing.[49] The SS doctor would make weekly inspections of the hospital. The Jewish doctor would provide a list of the sick, their prognosis and expected date of recovery and release. Selections followed and without exception a Jewish doctor would directly or indirectly participate in the selection process. He or she either advised on the patients' health, which would directly influence who the SS doctor selected. On other occasions the doctor was given a quota,[50] for example,

---

A Blockschreiber (block clerk or registrar) had to give the reports at roll call, as well as the food and death reports. Depending on the national composition of the block, many block elders needed interpreters for their work. The Schreibstube (administrative office) was headed by the Rapportschreiber (report writer); initially this was Paul Kozwara, then Gustav Herzog and finally Stefan Lembke. Here the prisoners were registered and the prisoner index managed, the prisoners assigned to blocks and the transport lists written when inmates had been selected for 'transfer' to Birkenau, generally meaning death in the gas chamber. Work in the administrative office also yielded the extremely risky opportunity to remove prisoners from selection lists or transpose record cards, in order to save individual prisoners. The report writer was responsible to the SS-man serving as Rapportführer (roll-call leader) and also to the camp elder (Grünberg, 2007)

49 The Auschwitz self-depended upon radically diminished feeling, upon ones not experiencing psychologically what one was doing. Lifton called this 'psychic numbing', a general category of diminished capacity or inclination to feel. Psychic numbing involves an interruption in psychic action. – in the creation and continuous re-creation of images and forms that constitutes the symbolizing or "formative process" characteristic of human mental life. The key function of numbing in the Auschwitz self is the avoidance of feelings of guilt when one is involved in killing. The Auschwitz self can then engage in medicalized killing, an ultimate form of numbered violence (Lifton 2000, 442).

50 In the case of quotas this may occur when a new train arrives with sick or injured prisoners who are considered potentially fit to work in the camps or the SS or Kapos supply the names of prisoners healthy or not to be murdered to prevent the doctors and nurses from hiding or

100 patients, and they would be required to provide the names to the SS doctor or the Blockältester. These patients were then administered phenol in the hospital or taken to be gassed. Lifton notes that killing by the phenol injection was institutionalized during the early phases of Auschwitz. The patient was taken to a treatment room and there administered a drug by a doctor or his assistant, who wore a white coat. In camp jargon this was referred to as 'spritzen' (to inject, squirt, spray), or being 'abgespritzt' (to be injected off or killed).

> Initially, phenol was injected into a victim's vein, maximizing the medical aura of the entire procedure ... Before long, the technique was changed to injecting the phenol directly into the heart. Some witnesses thought that the change was made because the veins were sometimes hard to locate, but the real reason seems to have been the greater killing efficiency of a direct cardiac injection. Patients injected by vein might linger for minutes or even an hour or more ... The 'concentrated aqueous solution of phenol' that was developed proved 'inexpensive, easy to use and absolutely effective when introduced into the heart ventricle', so that an injection of ten to fifteen millimetres (sic) into the heart caused death within fifteen seconds. (Lifton 2000, 254)

Lifton describes how phenol injections were given in Block 20:

> Two Jewish prisoner assistants brought a victim into the room (sometimes victims were brought in two at a time) and positioned him or her on a footstool, usually so that the right arm covered the victim's eyes and the left arm was raised sideways in a horizontal position ... The idea was for the victim's chest to be thrust out so that the cardiac area was maximally accessible for the lethal injection and for him or her to be unable to see what was happening ... The person giving the injection – most often the SDG Josef Klehr – filled his syringe from the bottle and then thrust the needle directly into the heart of the seated prisoner and emptied the contents of the syringe. (Lifton 2000, 254)

The practical and administrative processing of the killings was organized and structured down to minutiae. Once the selections were made, the administration clerk of the Schreibstube (Hospital administration), most likely Jewish,[51] would prepare death certificates and other relevant documentation for the camp command. Meticulous records were required to be kept by both the SS

---

protecting prisoners from selections. Initially the personal and moral pain of the prisoner doctor would be unimaginable when forced to meet a quota of names to be murdered. Later it will be argued that if and when a prisoner doctor carried out these horrendous duties in such a robotic fashion, it no longer constituted a dilemma.

51 The SS considered Jews as better educated and had greater language skills. This particularly applied to Western European Jews. The ability to speak several languages especially German, French, Polish and in 1944 Hungarian was an advantage. It is ironic that although the Nazis considered the Jews sub-human the former relied on the Jews to perform important functions in the camp.

and prisoner doctor although most were falsified. Records were kept including fever charts, orders for medicines, death books outlining cause of death, surgery reports and other medical documents, all concise and seemingly professional. Lily Hoenig, who worked in the Schreibstube, recalled, 'our supervisor, checked everything and returned it to me if so much as the dot of an 'i' was out of place or missing' (Shelley 1986, 88). Documents were signed by the Lagerarzt and distributed to several departments. Each file comprised the following.

a) A report of the death in eight copies sent to all interested administration departments of the headquarters.

b) A report sent to headquarters in four copies that included all personal data of the deceased.

c) A doctor's report in four copies that included description of the illness, the diagnosis, treatment and direct cause of death. From the beginning to the end the reports were completely falsified. They relied on the imagination of people who prepared the health records. To handle the ever -increasing death toll and death certificate numbers each individual scribe became a specialist in each individual disease. For example, one scribe was a specialist in heart disease another lung disease, another brain etc. In other cases, the scribes were provided with a list of diseases from which they could choose the cause of death.

d) A doctor's certificate in four copies. This particular certificate was issued without the prisoner's number.

e) The certificate confirming the death of the prisoner. This copy was for the registry department of births and deaths and included official personal data (Fejkiel 1994, 30).

At the trial of Rudolf Höss, Dr Jan Olbrycht testified, after examining the documents produced by the hospital administration:

> Had Nazism not been defeated, an impartial observer studying medical histories of Auschwitz prisoners and the protocols of their medical treatment might have come to the conclusion that sanitation, hygiene, and medical procedures in Auschwitz were exemplary and that medical care given to prisoners conformed to the latest guidelines of medical science and craft. (Olbrycht 1945)

The detail in the medical and death records would suggest that the SS were following normal civilized medical procedures and that their system operated with some legitimacy. However, research on medical records and survivors' testimonies show that little, if any, reliance can be placed on accuracy or legitimacy of the contents. Ironically both SS and prisoner doctors falsified medical records.

The former falsified the records and death certificates where a prisoner was murdered. In such cases, and there were hundreds of thousands, the cause of death of the prisoner was given a nominated medical illness or disease. In the case of the prisoner doctor, records were falsified to hide symptoms, such as high fevers, to keep the prisoner alive, even if only for a brief period. Although, why doctors would hide a prisoner's high fever, which might indicate the onset of a contagious disease and lead to epidemics and wholesale death from illness or mass murder, is a mystery. One would expect those prisoners most threatening to the health and welfare of all prisoners would be the first to be sacrificed.

The prisoners who worked in the Schreibstube were mainly Western European Jews, as they were considered better educated and more likely to be multi-lingual. As previously mentioned each clerk had a list of diseases and illnesses from which to choose and notate one as the cause of death. In most cases, medical records (ärztliche Berichte) showing the prisoner's gradual declining health were attached to the death certificate. These included heart rate, blood pressure and temperature charts and blood tests. At his trial Höss (Auschwitz-Birkenau State Museum, 1945) testified that the most popular causes of death were heart attack (Herzschlag), acute circulation insufficiency (Kreislauffinsuffizienz), pulmonary oedema with atrophy of the heart muscle, (Lungenödem bei Herzmuskeldegeneration), pulmonary inflammation (Lungenentzündung) or blood poisoning (Allgemeine Sepsis). Frieda Sender, a clerk in the Schreibstube, stated that they were required to write lists of names, birth dates and places of birth and causes of death but that many of the latter were not to be believed. For instance, quite frequently the cause of death for a little girl was given as 'weakness due to old age' (Shelley 1991, 82). Wieslaw Kielar, who also worked on writing death certificates (Totenmeldungen) in the Schreibstube, noted the following:

> Each deceased prisoner had to have a case history – which was fictional, of course. The camp administration demanded this and ordered me to do it. At first even when I knew a prisoner had been shot, I entered Herzschlag (heart attack), but I later realized that, if there were too many of these 'heart attacks' and Politische noticed, things might turn out badly for me. I therefore wrote the kind of Totenmeldungen that they wanted: I wrote Durchfall (diarrhoea) for a prisoner who had been shot, and Herzschlag for one who died of Durchfall, Nierentzündung for those who received a fatal injection and so on. In short, this was the perfidious falsification of the death certificates, camouflaging the mass murder committed against defenceless prisoners. (Kielar, n.d)

According to these records, fifty per cent died from heart disease including the 18-year-old Heinz Blut and 20 years old Jacob Lewkowioz. Over thirty per cent of the cohort died from lung disease. The entry of 'lung oedema at heart failure' can only have been made by someone deliberately inserting false detail or by someone with no idea of what they were inserting as a reason for death. We know that in the case of

Table 2: Death from suspected fabricated illnesses.

Name	DOB	D.O. Arrival	D.O. Death	Period in Camp	Age	Illness
Eduard Klubski	04.10.1918	16.10.1941	04.11.1941	3 weeks	23	Bauchfellentzündung: Peritonitis
Symcha Liberbon	20.07.1893	24.10.1941	04.11.1941	2 weeks	48	Gehirnschlag: Brain injury
Ezrael Merkin	20.12.1914	16.10.1941	06.11.1941	3 weeks	27	Rippenfellentzündung: Pleurisy
Abram Rosenzwajg	02.05.1897	24.10.1941	04.11.1941	2 weeks	44	Myocardinsuffiziens: Heart disease
Aleeksander Bednarezuk	17.11.1892	25.04.1941	06.11.1941	20 weeks	49	Herzwassersucht: Heart attack
Arnold Torner	28.11.1895	24.10.1942	06.11.1941	2 weeks	46	Myocardinsuffiziens: Heart disease
Abram Rubin	07.12.1899	16.10.1941	07.11.1941	3 weeks	42	Myocardinsuffiziens: Heart disease
Heinz Blut	04.09.1923	24.10.1941	07.11.1941	4 weeks	18	Versagen des Herzens und Kreislaufes: Heart attack
Kopel Brzezinski	22.04.1911	25.10.1941	07.11.1941	3 weeks	30	Herzwassersucht: Heart attack
Abram Glezman	16.11.1907	01.10.1941	06.11.1941	4 weeks	24	Herzmuskelschwäche: weakening of heart muscles
Jacob Lewowioz	12.06.1921	16.10.1941	06.11.1941	3 weeks	20	Versagen des Herzens und Kreislaufes: Heart attack
Szlama Hubarman	12.08.1922	01.10.1941	06.11.1941	5 weeks	19	Herzwassersucht: Heart attack
Samul Frydman	15.06.1913	25.10.1941	06.11.1941	2 weeks	28	Lungentuberkuloseo: Tuberculosis
Karl Mautner	13.12.1894	31.10.1941	04.11.1941	1 weeks	47	Lungenödem: Lung disease
Abram Kwiat	01.10.1914	24.10.1941	04.11.1941	2 weeks	27	Lungenödem: Lung disease
Ozkar Lanzar	26.07.1908	24.10.1941	06.11.1941	2 weeks	33	Lungenödem: Lung disease

(continued)

Table 2: (continued)

Name	DOB	D.O. Arrival	D.O. Death	Period in Camp	Age	Illness
Leon Anderman	25.12.1896	22.10.1941	06.11.1941	2 weeks	46	Lungenödem: Lung disease
Chil Zyibberman	25.08.1909	15.09.1941	06.11.1941	7 weeks	32	Lungentuberkuloseo: Tuberculosis

Courtesy of the Auschwitz Museum and ITS

Hans Redlich, prisoner 43798, who was shot 'while fleeing', the cause of death was recorded as plötzlicher Tod, sudden death, implying a heart attack. These prisoners were in Auschwitz for a very short time, some only one or two weeks. How many were in fact beaten to death, executed between Block 10 and Block 11, or admitted to hospital but died from phenol injections? How did Aleeksander Bednarezuk really die? He was in Auschwitz for twenty weeks. Did he become a Muselmänn and die of a heart attack or was he killed by injection or by a bullet? Did Symcha Liberbon have a stroke or did he suffer brain damage and die from a beating? The endemic fraud and deception in the medical system is a warning to researchers of Nazi medicine. Apart from testimony by prisoners who worked in the system and survived there is no credible evidence or documentation of what truly took place. It was only in name that the hospital and infirmaries could in any way be called part of a health system; rather, they were fundamental to an extermination system.

At this stage of the war Germany was enjoying success on the battlefield and the prospect of a never-ending supply of slave labour. They could afford to kill as many Jews as possible. Would these Jews have been murdered if it were 1943 when Germany needed every fit person available for slave labour? In September 1942, a new SS Standortarzt was appointed to Auschwitz, SS Hauptsturmführer Dr Eduard Wirths, who had a significant impact on the health system and conditions in the camp. According to Langbein (2004) and Dr Wladyslaw Fejkiel (1994), the atmosphere within the hospital system changed upon Wirths' arrival. Wirth brought with him to the camp a few dozen Austrian and German communists who had worked with him as nurses in Dachau concentration camp.

> These inmates were favoured by the SS garrison physician, who was a Nazi but hated criminals with an elemental passion. The new arrivals quickly familiarised themselves with the Auschwitz atmosphere, established contact with the group of Polish democrats, and with the aid of the SS garrison physician produced a sort of revolt in the infirmaries. (Langbein 2004, 370)

Fejkiel testified that he considered Wirths 'an intelligent physician and not a bad person. He brought medicines and knew how to combat typhus' (Langbein 2004, 371), whereas Wirth's predecessor had fought typhus by having the lice gassed together with the patients. According to Fejkiel, although Wirth was a Nazi and carried out orders as such, taking part in selections in the hospitals and on the arrival ramps, he did take action to eradicate diseases such as typhus, stopped the killing by phenol injection, reduced the number of prisoners sent to Block 11, and closed some of the more horrendous torture cells. According to Langbein (2004, 379), 'if the mortality rate in 1943 had remained as high as it was in the summer of 1942, before Wirths came to Auschwitz, it would have been necessary to register 93,000 more deaths.'

Despite the camp's objective to provide labour, Auschwitz continued as a vast industrial death factory. It was operated as a sophisticated human production line and anyone deemed unable or unsuitable to work was considered waste material and murdered or allowed to starve or freeze to death. They were regarded as no more than a part of a machine or engine that was discarded and destroyed when it failed to function.

5 Block 10

Jewish Doctors and Human Experimentation

When all that we know, or feel, or see,
Shall pass like an unreal mystery.
Percy Shelley (1907)

Dr Aliza Barouch, a doctor who entered Block 10 as a human guinea pig and later became a doctor working in the block recalled:

> Gradually we found out that Block 10 was an experimental block and that we women were to be used as guinea pigs. Two of the main experimenters were Clauberg and Schumann ... Both of them tortured the girls: they removed their virginity, irradiated and sterilized them, removed their ovaries and contaminated them with cancer. They violated and disfigured their bodies and transformed them into eunuchs. (Shelley 1991)

Block 10 was synonymous with evil. From 1942 until the liquidation of the camp, it was the centre of pseudoscientific human medical experiments that arguably represented an enormous violation of medical ethics[52] and the Hippocratic Oath in history. In Block 10, hundreds of young women underwent radiotherapy treatment and operations as part of a sterilization program the Nazis believed would support their demographic and racial policies, and for the immediate future solve labour supply problems. The women were human guinea pigs subjected to unscientific and unethical medical experiments. Women as shown in Fig. 17., were tied to examination beds for scientific medical experiments often left dying from infections. The aim was to devise a method that would secretly and efficiently sterilize as many women as possible in the shortest period. According to Dr Karel Sperber, another Jewish doctor who worked in Block 10, the women were exposed to damaging doses of X-rays until their ovaries became sterile. To confirm the experiments were successful, Clauberg removed the ovaries by an abdominal operation. The women lived as long as they were useful. In most cases, they were murdered once the experiments had been carried out and the results were known.

SS doctor Adolf Pokorny wrote to Heinrich Himmler explaining the rationale behind the experiments as follows:

> If we are able to discover as quickly as possible the means that could imperceptibly cause sterilization in a relatively short period of time, then we will have acquired a new,

---

[52] At the time of WWII ethics did not have a great presence in medical research. Ironically Germany was the first country to introduce a code of ethics for medical research. The first code was introduced in 1900 and this was revised in 1933. It is argued that the 1900 code of ethics was more demanding than the Nuremberg Code of Ethics established after the war.

https://doi.org/10.1515/9783110598216-009

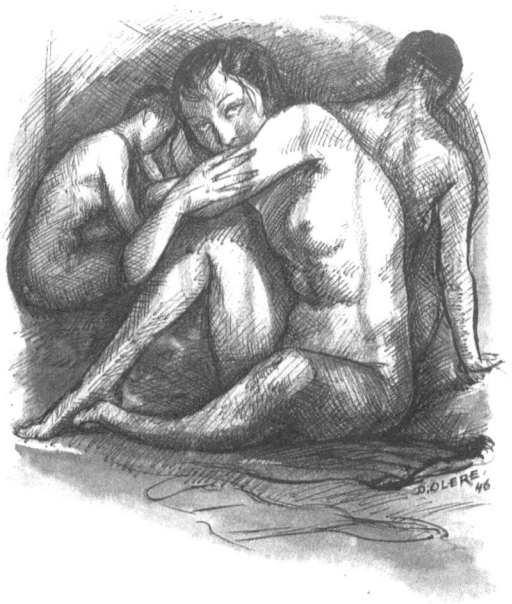

Fig. 16: Young girls used as human guinea pigs. Olere (1989)

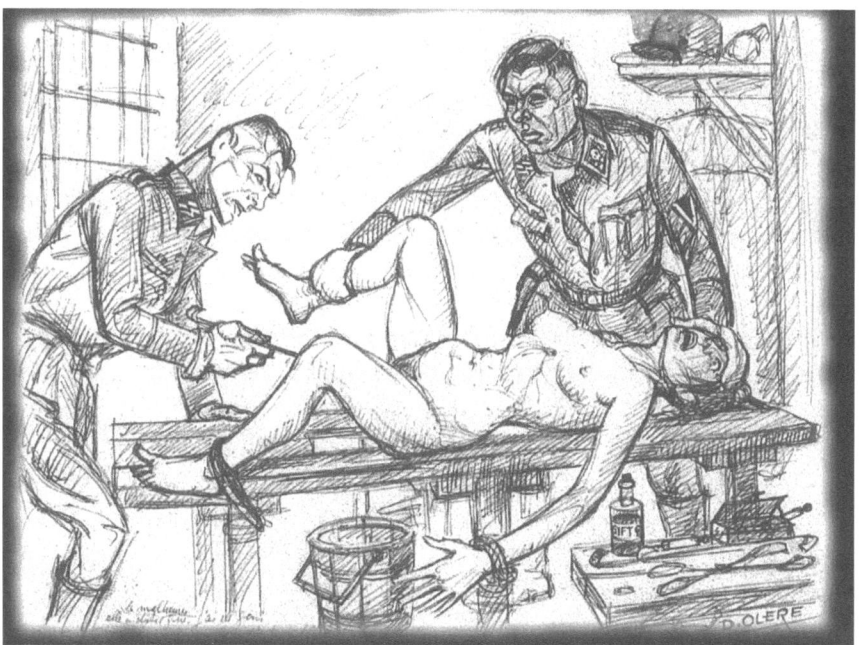

Fig. 17: Young women underwent radiotherapy treatment and operations as part of a steriliza-tion program. Olere and Oler (1998, 59)

effective weapon. The broad possibilities are alone suggested by the thought that three million Bolsheviks currently held as prisoners could be sterilized, and as a result, they would stand at our disposal as workers, but without the ability to multiply. (Mitscherlich & Mielke 1949, p. 237)

He was not alone in his opinion. SS Oberführer Viktor Brack[53] agreed:

Among the ten million Jews in Europe are, I figure, at least two to three millions of men and women, who are fit enough for work. Considering the extraordinary difficulties, the labour problem presents us with, I hold the view that these two to three million should be specifically selected and preserved. This can however only be done, if at the same time they are rendered incapable to propagate. (USHMM Archives Doc 205 in RG 30.001M)

In July 1942, Karl Brandt as chief SS doctor recorded a summary of a meeting held in respect to the sterilization of Jewesses. The following is a translation of the memorandum giving Clauberg permission to commence research in Auschwitz on how to effectively and secretly sterilize millions of Jews:

Führer – Headquarters July 1942
Top Secret
1 copy

On 7 July 1942, a discussion took place between the Reichführer SS, SS Brigadeführer Professor Dr Gebhardt, SS Brigadeführer Glücks and SS Brigadeführer Clauberg, Königshütte.

Topic of the discussion was the sterilization of Jewesses. The Reichsführer has promised SS-Brigadeführer Professor Clauberg that the Auschwitz concentration camp will be at his disposal for his experiments on human beings and animals. By means of some fundamental experiments a method should be found which would lead to sterilization without their knowledge. The Reichsführer SS wanted to get another report as soon as the results of these experiments would become known, so that the sterilization of Jewesses could then be carried out in actuality. It should also be examined, preferably in cooperation with Professor Dr Hohlfelder an X-ray specialist in Germany, in what way sterilization of men could be achieved by X-ray treatment. The Reichsführer SS called the special attention of all gentlemen present to the fact that the matter

---

53 Brack was responsible for organising and implementing the T4 killings. He participated in the first trial killing in Brandenburg in January 1940. Up to 1943 Brack was also involved in other euthanasia crimes such as the murder of concentration prisoners in Action 14F13 in the death camps in Poland as part of Aktion Reinhard as well as in attempts to castrate people using x-rays in Auschwitz-Birkenau.

involved was most secret and should be discussed only with the officers in charge and that the persons present at the experiments or discussions had to pledge secrecy.

(Signature) Brandt
(USHMM Archives Doc 216 in RG 30.00M)

Clauberg commenced his experiments in late 1942 in Block 30[54] in Birkenau and from April 1943 in Block 10 in the main camp. Block 10 was persona non grata and the windows of the two-storied brick building were blacked-out so that no one could see in or out of the block (Shelley 1991, 8).[55] The upper floor comprised of accommodation for four hundred prisoners occupying two large wards. The prisoners were separated depending on the type of experiment – sterilization, cancer of the uterus and blood transfusions. The ground floor accommodated the living quarters of prisoner doctors, nurses and auxiliary staff, the operating theatres and laboratories, dark room and guard quarters. The prisoners were given bigger food portions, better clothing and slept in beds but lived in constant fear of the radiation and surgery and the of selections. In a statement after the war Dr Margita Schwalbova, a Jewish doctor working in Block 10, describes the experiments and the suffering of the women:

> These human guinea pigs knew through the nursing personnel and through rumors that they were used for sterilization experiments or for artificial insemination. Both of these possibilities filled them with fear. Insemination would have meant a death sentence. (Shelley 1991, 14)

SS-Untersturmführer Dr Hans Münch, who arrived in Block 10 in the autumn or winter of 1943, was told that 'as bearers of secrets (Geheimnisträger) they [the

---

54 Block 30 was a wooden barrack and belonged to the Revier (hospital complex). Inside there was a bedroom for prisoners, a waiting room and an adjacent room with two Siemens x-ray apparatuses. Across from these machines, there was a small booth, insulated with lead plates for protection from radiation, with glass windows from where Schumann could operate the x-ray apparatuses (Shelley 1991, 21).

55 The first guinea pigs to arrive were one hundred Greek Jewesses with prison numbers 41,500 to 41,600. In April 1943 another transport of one hundred and ten women was admitted to Block 10 (42,500 to 42600). On June 29, 1943, the patient pool increased by sixty-five women from Berlin, with numbers around 47,400 and on July 21, seventy women from France with numbers around 50,300 were added. Subsequently, three transports from the Netherlands followed – forty women with numbers around 56,000 in August and one hundred women on September 16 and 23, 1943, with numbers around 62,400 and 63,100 respectively. Dr Wirth selected the women for Block 10 (Shelley 1991, 8).

women prisoners in Block 10] had to be gassed' (Shelley 1991, 277) Dr Karel Sperber, a Jewish doctor who also worked in Block 10 and witnessed the work of Clauberg, confirms this:

> But something I do know; after the inmates of the experimental station had served their purpose they were blessed with the mercy of a quick death by cyanide gas in the gas chambers of Birkenau. (Sperber 1946)

Although there were some SS doctors who carried out experiments in Block 10, the block became known as Claubergs' Block. Clauberg and Schumann were involved in sterilisation with the former experimenting with Jewish women while the latter specialised in irradiation and castration of men. Wirths, the medical superintendent, researched pre-cancerous growths of the uterus by surgically removing the cervix. Bruno Weber, director of the Hygiene Institute, carried out experiments on blood. In their capacity as surgeons and researchers, prisoner doctors participated to some degree in experiments. Jewish doctor Dr Anna Seemanowa assisted world-renowned Jewish bacteriologist Dr Ludwick Fleck and his wife Ernestina Waldmann in Block 10 in their work to diagnose syphilis, typhus, spotted fever, malaria and other illnesses using serological tests. Both Jewish and non-Jewish prisoner doctors worked with SS doctors. Dering, a Polish surgeon, earned notoriety for collaborating with the Nazi doctors while Dr Hautval, a female German surgeon, earned praise and respect for defying Nazi orders and refusing under any circumstances to operate on patients. Both survived Auschwitz.

The lives of Jewish doctors and nurses in Block 10 were paradoxical. In the first instance, the doctors were afforded reasonable conditions. They received adequate food, clothing and accommodation and, most importantly, they were not subject to roll calls or the extremes of the weather. The working facilities and equipment were relatively modern and medical supplies and medications adequate. On the other hand, the environment in which they worked was a 'sort of nightmare, that was a mixture of hell and a lunatic asylum' (Lorska 1971, 81). Situational factors and personal circumstances led the prisoner doctor to react in different ways. The case studies of Drs Alina Brewda and Maximilian Samuel bear this point out. Brewda was regarded as an independent individual who commanded the respect of her patients, colleagues and SS doctors and who worked courageously to comfort and protect patients. By contrast, Samuel, a world-renowned gynaecologist and pioneer of detecting precancerous growths on the cervix, was criticized and even condemned by colleagues and historians for allegedly collaborating with SS doctors by operating on Jewish women in sterilisation experiments.

Dr Alina Brewda

Alina Brewda was born in Warsaw on 13 June 1905.[56] Her family included her mother, father and an older brother. Both parents were dentists and, their surgeries adjoined the family home. Alina's father was Jewish though not very observant while her mother's family had converted to Christianity. Despite this, Alina's mother insisted on maintaining a Jewish home.

> All in all it was a very happy childhood. My parents used to take us to the theatre, to concerts and to the ballet, and we went to the cinema every week...we also went for drives in a hired carriage drawn by two large, handsome horses. We drove down the fashionable Aleje Ujardowskie with its lovely lime trees, to the Larienki gardens with its open-air theatre by the lake, and onto the charming chateau of Belvedere. (Minney 1966, 14)

Alina had a loving, secure and close relationship with her parents. She considered herself more similar to her mother, who was resourceful and had a robust, energetic constitution, than to her father, who was soft, kind and gentle. Some of the characteristics inherited from both parents were to have a significant influence in Auschwitz. From an early age, Brewda participated in athletics; she loved climbing trees and going on cross-country walks. Despite the happy and vibrant surroundings, she was stubborn and dominating from an early age:

> I was not a very likeable child...I was always blunt and outspoken and by temperament extremely bossy. Although I was generally the youngest and smallest among a group of children, I automatically took charge and, surprisingly, even the boys accepted my lead, and allowed me to make the decisions and to organize everything. (Minney 1966, 13)

Because of her stubbornness, she was sent to pre-school at the age of two, but this was not successful because of sickness. Instead, she received private tutoring until the age of eight. She then attended a Russian school rather than a Polish school as the former gave her a better opportunity to enter university. After graduating from secondary school in 1923, Alina went to Paris to perfect her French, and to London for a short period. She returned home to begin her medical studies at the University of Warsaw.

Her early childhood and adolescence were free of overt antisemitism, and it appears there was a healthy relationship with non-Jewish friends. It was during her years at university that Brewda first experienced antisemitism. This exposure was distressing, and she felt humiliated and hurt. The Students' Medical

---

56 At that time the state of Poland did not exist, and Warsaw was a Russian city that was the headquarters of the Russian Governor-General.

Association stripped her of her membership. During class, she and her fellow Jewish students were discriminated against, particularly when they were refused permission to dissect Christian cadavers. The students were required to receive permission from their rabbi to use Jewish corpses for their clinical research and education. Even worse was the threat of violence:

> A large number of two hundred and twenty Christian medical students, after arming themselves with sticks fitted with razor blades, lay in wait for the twenty-five Jewish students and set about them in the dissection room and operating theatre. (Minney 1966, 18)

Despite the obstacles and the challenges, Brewda was determined to complete her studies. In 1930, at the age of twenty-five, she graduated and commenced work as a doctor at the Wolsky General hospital. Since her work at the hospital was unpaid, she lived with her parents. To gain more experience in gynaecology, she left for Paris in 1931. There she joined L'Hôpital Bretenneau and worked with Professor Marcel Metzgar, a world-renowned specialist in gynecology, and then moved to the Bocca-Hospital to work with Professor Jean-Louis Faure, another famous gynaecologist. It was her training with such eminent specialists that led Brewda to Block 10 where she would work on experiments on women. In 1932 Brewda returned to Warsaw where significant social and political changes were taking place that would eventually end in disaster for the Polish Jews. In the years up until 1939, she travelled abroad, established a private practice in Warsaw as a gynaecologist and obstetrician and worked in a small Jewish obstetric hospital. She couldn't find work in the larger hospitals because of the imposition of quotas on the number of Jewish doctors allowed to work in hospitals. With the invasion and occupation of Poland, Brewda became another member of the Warsaw ghetto that eventually held over five hundred thousand Jews. Life in the ghetto was difficult. The appalling conditions were a breeding ground for disease, and Brewda with other doctors were fighting a losing battle against epidemics. Professor Ludwik Hirszfeld[57] recalls,

> Everywhere in front of the houses lay piles of rubbish and excrement, sometimes reaching the level of the second floor. Rubbish-disposal did not function in the Jewish section...owing to the frosts and the lack of fuel, the sewer pipes were often damaged. As a result heaps of excrement were lying in the streets, in the courtyards, on the staircases, and even the floors of the apartments. (Minney 1966, 39)

---

[57] Luwik Hirszfeld was a Jewish Polish microbiologist and a scientist. He converted to Catholicism. He was a prominent scientist and academic in Warsaw; however, after the occupation of Poland by Germany he lost his post as director of the State Hygiene Institute of Warsaw. He was considered a 'non-Aryan' and lived in the Warsaw ghetto.

In April 1943 Brewda was sent to Majdanek[58] concentration camp:

> The journey took twenty-four hours during which they had no food or drink. There was no lavatory either. Cramped though they were, some of the passengers with difficulty hacked away at the floor of the train to make holes for use as an outlet, but few were able to reach them. Many died during the journey. (Minney 1966, 76)

At the camp Brewda came to the attention of Dr Rindfleisch, who was head doctor of the camp. Rindfleisch instructed her to establish a hospital for prisoners with typhus.

> I had by now – six weeks after my arrival – a staff of eleven Jewish doctors and seventy-four Jewish nurses...I set up a hospital for the Russian women. I had bunks put up for them and got straw for use in the mattresses. I was even able to get sheets and blankets from the stores. (Minney 1966, 87)

Her work was so satisfactory that SS Standartenführer, Dr Enno Lolling, Deputy Inspector-General of medical services of concentration camps, requisitioned her to Auschwitz. Brewda knew of Auschwitz and resisted, naively insisting on certain conditions: firstly, that she would not have her head shaved; secondly, that she would not be tattooed; and thirdly, that she would not be sent to the gas chambers if she were unable to continue her work. Lolling acceded but his assurances were hollow. Although her head was not shaved, she was tattooed. In regard to being spared execution, she would learn when she was sent to the dreaded Block 11,[59] the punishment block, that no Jew was untouchable. She believed she would be working in the female hospital but was appointed head doctor of Block 10 under the direct orders of Dr Eduard Wirths. This gave her what she felt to be sufficient authority to challenge even the SS. If SS guards showed her disrespect by addressing her in the familiar 'du' rather than 'Sie', she would

---

58 Majdanek was a Nazi concentration camp established on the outskirts of the city of Lublin. Although initially purposed for forced labor rather than extermination, the camp was used to kill people on an industrial scale during Operation Reinhard, the German plan to murder all Jews within their General Government territory of Poland
59 This block situated in the Stammlager (Auschwitz I main camp) was intended solely to punish prisoners through torture. Between the tenth and eleventh block stood the death wall (reconstructed after the war) where thousands of prisoners were lined up for execution by firing squad. The block contained special torture chambers in which various punishments were applied to prisoners. Some could include being locked in a dark chamber for several days, while others were punished to stand in four standing cells. In these special compartments (one square metre each, with a hole 5x5 cm for breathing), four prisoners had to remain standing (for lack of space) night after night for several and up to twenty days as punishment; while being forced to continue working during daytime.

admonish them 'I am not "du" to you...Remember I'm "Frau Doktor" to you, as I am to Dr Wirths. If any of you try to beat me or ill-treat me, I'll have you thrown out of the Block' (Shelley, 1991, 33). This response was indicative of the same confidence, assertiveness and self-esteem that allowed her to question the cruel and painful operations conducted by Polish and SS doctors. However, such bravado put her at risk of punishment and perhaps was the reason why she was ultimately incarcerated in Block 11.

Within a short period of arriving in Block 10, Brewda discovered what was happening under the guise of medicine:

> I made a practice of going upstairs at least once a day. The Greek girls seemed terribly afraid to say anything ... after some days some of them told me ... they were suffering from burns. I examined them and found that these were due to deep X-ray radiation. The burns were raw. I asked the girls about them and they told me they had been taken into a dark room and come out with these burns ... after examining the scars and the burns closely I realised the girls had probably had irradiation of the ovaries and that a pretty strong dose had been given them without proper care and skill. Their skin was covered with suppurating blisters and ulcers ... I did what I could for them. (Minney 1966, 120)

As a gynaecologist, what she witnessed was abhorrent to her. Although Lolling had guaranteed she would not be punished if she refused to work in the camp and could possibly return to the previous camp, she felt her duty as a doctor to the prisoners was more important than her own well-being. She never tested the guarantee. Although she worked with Wirths and Clauberg, Brewda indicated she did not become involved in the experiments. Both doctors shrouded their experiments in a cloud of secrecy, and Brewda recalled:

> I had been especially instructed by Dr Wirths to stay away from his guinea pigs. I only knew that they (Jewish women) had a caustic fluid injected into their uterus' while, simultaneously, x-rays were taken to ascertain the blockage. The pain caused by these sterilization experiments must have been tremendous, and the screams of the women could be heard throughout the whole block. Sometimes, even the SS women came to me and asked what Clauberg was doing to these women to make them scream so horribly. (Shelley, 1991, 38)

However, it was Brewda's dealings with Schumann and a Polish prisoner doctor, Wladslaw Dering, that caused her the most anguish and torment. Schumann wanted her to perform operations to remove prisoners' ovaries and Brewda refused. She was outraged at the pain and suffering of the patients and uselessness of the operations and procedures. Out of fear for the patients, her nurturing instinct and professional ethics forced her to try and intervene in some of the operations and procedures carried out by both doctors. In one case she recalls,

As I entered I heard a girl screaming and the Greek word for mother was clearly audible. I went with Dr Schumann into the anteroom of the operating theatre and saw one of the Greek girls from my Block (Block 10) being held down on a special table by two male prisoners in white coats – the girl was held in a suitable position to receive a spinal injection. She kept on screaming ... Dr Dering was there too, washing his hands at a basin. Dr Schumann asked me to calm the girls and left me in the anteroom with the Greek girls, the two male prisoners in white coats and Dr Dering ... the door of the theatre was open and I saw a girl lying strapped to the operating-table. I went up to Dr Dering and said: 'Do you realize that these girls have had irradiation quite recently?' He said 'I know,' I asked him what he was doing, he said, 'Ovariectomies'. He then went into the theatre and I followed because the girl on the operating table was screaming and crying and trying to release herself. Dr Dering put on his gloves and the table was tilted to form an angle of about thirty degrees, with the patient's head downwards, which is the lithotomy position. I sat on a stool by the girl's head and tried to comfort her. I realised now what was being done to her and I knew that she would be able to see the removal of her ovary because it would be reflected in the operating lamp ... Dr Dering then proceeded to make abdominal incisions, and told me to keep the girl quiet. I told him 'What do you think you are doing? This is a young girl, she has already had irradiation of the ovary, so why do you have to operate?' He did not reply. He cut the peritoneum, and used forceps to lift up the uterus. He then put the forceps between the tube and the ovary and cut off the ovary – one only – and put it in a specimen basin beside him. The operation took about ten minutes. I had never seen this done so quickly before ... the girl was then carried out on a stretcher by the two male prisoners and Dr Dering went and gave the spinal injection to the next girl, who also began to scream ... he performed a similar operation on the second girl. (Minney 1966, 128)

Brewda was racked with anxiety and fear for the victim both from a human and professional viewpoint. Although unable to prevent the operations, Brewda at least voiced her disapproval. Dering claimed he was in fear of his life if he did not co-operate, 'I have my orders. They will kill me. I have to do it' (Minney 1966, 129). Yet Hautval, who like Dering was non-Jewish, was not punished when she refused to carry out operations. Was Dering antisemitic to the extent that he had no qualms about or even willingly participated in the operations? His behaviour and treatment of Jewish prisoners certainly did not suggest compassion or empathy. Witnesses at the famous libel trial brought by Dering against the author Leon Uris and the publisher of the book Exodus in 1964, reveal the extraordinary ethical and humane gulf between the doctors Dering and Brewda. One witness at the trial told of the comfort and care Brewda gave her:

Because of the pains I shouted, screamed, and they took me to another room, put me on a table. There was a kind of screen before my face. There was a big lamp. I saw the reflections in the lamp. I felt they were doing something but did not realize what. Dr Brewda was there. She put her hand on my cheek and consoled me. Then she said, 'N'aie pas peur, mon enfant.' I understood a little French and I knew it meant 'Don't be afraid, my child' and she added, 'It will pass quickly'. (Minney 1966, 131)

Lucy Chimino from Saloniki, Greece, confirms this in her description of her own ordeal as a guinea pig in the infamous block:

> They performed anaesthesia in Block 21, which was opposite to Block 10. They took us there on a stretcher; they transferred us to this place. We were waiting in line, in the meanwhile there was somebody there who put our head between his legs and our body was bent over, he gave us an injection for anaesthesia in our spine, half of our bodies were anaesthetised. Each of us went into the operating room. There was a woman doctor in the operating room who always patted our heads, she said do not be afraid, it will be alright.... (Chimino 1984)

Despite the glowing testimonials from ex-patients, Brewda did not escape criticism. Ima Spanjaar, a Jewish nurse recalls the following:

> [Brewda] lived in luxury. I remember one evening after 6 pm ... I had to ask something of Dr Brewda and knocked on the door of her little room. She was dining with two or three others. The table was elegantly set with a white tablecloth and delicate china dishes (white with pink flowers). There was a tantalizing fragrance of good food, animated conversation and rosy colored cheeks. Dr Brewda suddenly became furious at me for having glanced at this concealed corrupt opulence. (Shelley 1986, 51)

Brewda was no doubt enjoying being able to share food and conversation with a select few, features of life as it once was, and to feel human again. It was probably a form of affirmation of the self. Yet it demonstrated that Brewda was very much like any other prisoner in that, given the opportunity to enjoy better conditions, she would do so even at the expense of others. Ima recalled that Brewda would recite everyday 'to be or not to be' and 'Erst kommt das Fressen und dann kommt die Moral' (food first and morals later).[60] In late July 1944 Brewda was suddenly taken to Block 11, the punishment block:

> I was put into a minute cell with just a bunk and a tiny bucket for use as a toilet. There was no water at all. I had to take out the bucket once a day ... and wash it in a communal washroom ...for two days I was given nothing to eat or drink. (Shelley 1986, 40)

She had no indication of what had precipitated this punishment, however, it can be assumed that her antagonism and highhandedness toward fellow doctors and the SS played some part. It may have been to teach her a lesson and to make her insecure. It may have been to teach all prisoner doctors that they were not above punishment or free of uncertainty and fear. After seventeen days of solitary confinement she was released and transferred to Birkenau, where she worked as a seamstress for nearly four months, never knowing why she was put through the

---

60 The quote, literally, '*First comes the grub, then morality*', comes from *Brecht's Dreigroschenoper (The Threepenny Opera)*.

ordeal. In her words Birkenau was a 'hell hole' (Shelley 1986, 40). In December 1944 Brewda was assigned to the hospital in Birkenau. She continued to carry out abortions as she had in Block 10. 'I had been performing abortions on Jewish girls for I knew that all pregnant Jewesses were sent straight to the gas chamber' (Minney 1966, 160). On 18 January 1945, the Nazis began to evacuate the camp. Brewda, some nurses and a number of patients began the tortuous death march that would eventually take them to Ravensbrück, another death camp. The journey, first on foot and then in an open cattle train, subjected them to the worst conditions and the majority of prisoners died from exhaustion, froze to death, or were shot or beaten to death. Yet Brewda refused to give up or to leave her patients. The conditions once they got to Ravensbrück were appalling:

> No food at all was brought to us. We were given nothing either to eat or to drink. Our hunger became so unbearable that many left their bunks and let themselves out of the window to get at the snow, which they stuffed into their mouths. We were also covered with lice, all of us. There would inevitably have been an appalling epidemic of typhus, but we rubbed ourselves with snow to make ourselves clean and got rid of most of the lice this way. (Minney 1966, 189)

After a number of days Brewda was transferred to another concentration camp, Neustadt-Glewe, where she contracted typhus and became critically ill. She recovered and once again was placed in charge of one of the hospital huts. Conditions were similar to Auschwitz. Food and water was in short supply as were medical supplies and equipment. She recalls, 'There were about a dozen deaths a day' (Minney 1966, 191). She would not record these until twenty-four hours later so that the rations of the dead could be used to feed prisoners who were still alive. It was another nine weeks before Brewda was finally freed.

Little is known of her life after liberation except that she travelled to the United Kingdom. She lived in north London with her husband, an ex- Polish general, and worked in general practice.

Maximilian Samuel

Dr Maximilian Samuel[61] did not survive Auschwitz. He was murdered in late 1943 but it is not known on whose orders. Samuel was a controversial and important figure in the history of medicine in Auschwitz. To his colleagues he

---

61 This section owes much to the excellent work of Ruth Jolanda Weinberger in providing information on Samuel in her book Fertility Experiments in Auschwitz-Birkenau: Perpetrators and Their Victims (Weinberger 2009, 260–274).

was either a collaborator or a misguided fool who became increasingly senile and was convinced that by working with the SS doctors he would save his daughter's life? To many of the victims who after the war became pregnant give him due credit because of his betrayal of the SS doctors' orders to sterilize all Jewish women. To these women he was a hero. There is little agreement regarding his character or his behaviour between colleagues and patients.

The early life of Samuel is unknown. After exhaustive research, I found nothing of substance about the early life of this enigmatic Jewish man. He was born in Cologne in 1880, studied medicine and became a gynaecologist and academic in his home city. He was recognized as a leading surgeon. He served as a military doctor for Germany with distinction during the First World War. Despite this service neither he nor his family escaped the tentacles of Nazi policies towards the Jews. As with thousands of Jewish doctors and dentists, his licence was revoked. However, when given the opportunity to escape Germany, he refused. Like so many Jewish veterans, he thought he would be exempt from harsh treatment. He found this was not the case and he decided that he and his family should leave Germany. After a failed attempt by the Nazis to send Samuel and his family to a camp they escaped to Belgium. Samuel, his wife Nedzig and daughter Lieselotte were captured in Bruxelles and deported to France to be incarcerated in Belfort prison on the 27 August, 1942. On August 31, they departed Drancy transit camp for Auschwitz (ITS Archives, Transport list).

Archival records do not disclose anything of significance of Samuel's arrival at the camp, but it is certain that the train trip was horrendous and that the scene at the transit ramp was chaotic, humiliating and brutal. Tragically, on arrival, Samuel's wife was sent to the gas while Samuel and Lieselotte were selected for the labour camp. Samuel was over sixty, which would normally have condemned him to the gas chambers. The critical shortage of doctors saved his life. He was assigned to a factory clinic in Monowitz, and with the status of a doctor enjoyed better conditions. It is only an assumption but the status of privilege and the possibility that he and Lieselotte had contact may have given him the opportunity to provide her with additional food and better clothing. Samuel came to the attention of Mengele, who knew him as a gynaecologist and specialist surgeon, and he was reassigned to Block 10. Wirths was a competent researcher but he was not an experienced and skilled surgeon. There is no evidence but Mengele may have thought that Samuel, who was a respected surgeon, would make a good addition to the team working on sterilization experiments.[62] Both Clauberg and Schumann

---

62 Affidavit by Klempfner, July 27, 1946, NI-311 used in the deposition by Adelaide de Jong during the Belsen Trial (Philips 1949, 668). De Jong was sterilized by Dr Samuel.

had assured Himmler that through a sterilization program they could create a large workforce of two to three million Jews who could not procreate. Samuel and the Polish prisoner doctor Dering were charged with the task of removing the reproductive organs of women who had undergone severe X-ray irradiation, whereby 'large parts of the uterus, with one (and sometimes both) of the ovaries were excised and sent for examination, to observe the effectiveness of the irradiations' (Nadav 2009, 129). Both procedures, the irradiation and the surgery, were painful and often fatal. Samuel was also assigned to participate in questionable experiments into cervical cancer. They consisted of a procedure that involved the excision of cervices from women who had been treated against the spread of cancer. The cervix was photographed with the aid of a colposcope and tissue was sent to the Frauenklinik Altona (women's hospital) in Hamburg for examination.

A number of explanations have been proposed as to why Samuel supposedly worked with the SS. The most plausible is that he hoped to save the life of his daughter, who was in Birkenau. He reportedly wrote to Himmler asking him to spare her life on account of his services to Germany and the experimental work he had undertaken in Block 10. His appeal was either ignored or never reached Himmler. Samuel was put to death soon after. There is no evidence that Clauberg, Wirths, Schumann or Mengele made any agreement with Samuel regarding his daughter's life. The testimony of Wirths after 1945 did not reveal any agreement with Samuel that his daughter's life would be spared if he worked with the SS doctors. Little was known of him or the role he played until victims and colleagues gave evidence during the Dering libel trial[63] in London in 1963. Three prisoner doctors, Brewda, Hautval and Lorska testified, giving mostly damning evidence of Samuel's behaviour and competence. Lorska said, 'I was under the impression that what he was doing was not unpleasant for him' (Weinberger 2009, 263). Brewda conjectured that Samuel was blackmailed into working with the SS on the basis that it would save his daughter's life. Hautval considered that Samuel was driven by fear and the desire to satisfy the Nazis. She said,

> This became visible. And since he was Jewish, his situation was more dangerous than mine. Furthermore, it was said that his daughter was in the camp. Without a doubt, he told himself that by obeying his masters he could save himself. (Weinberger 2009, 263)

In 1962 Hautval took a softer view saying that she thought Samuel was a competent doctor, but that stress and pressure had gradually affected his mind and competence. Brewda remembered Samuel as 'an old man, in a very bad mental

---

63 Wladislaw Dering sued the writer Leon Uris over claims made in his novel Exodus that Dering had been involved in human medical experiments in Auschwitz.

condition and, I do not know, bewildered' (Weinberger 2009, 264). Lorska assessed him as an old man who in time became senile, that 'mentally he was not quite right', (Weinberger 2009, 264). Samuel's age undoubtedly had an impact on his mental state, particularly considering the stress he was under and the fear he felt both for his daughter and himself. Survivors paint a different picture of Samuel. Many survivors, who after the Holocaust went on to have families, credit Samuel. They provided testimony that Samuel did not perform the operation that he was meant to do. How else were they able to give birth? Perhaps Samuel was not as senile or befuddled as reported. Aliza Barouch was operated on by Samuels to have both ovaries removed (ovariectomies). She protested becoming hysterical, crying, 'I don't have a baby' (Shelley 1986, 82). Schumann produced a gun threatening Aliza 'you either go down or I shoot. Crawl like a dog and come down' (Shelley 1986, 82). She had no choice. After the operation, she found Samuel standing beside her bed stroking her head and he said to her, 'If you live, remember me' (Shelley 1986, 82). On Rosh Hashanah 1946 Aliza gave birth to a baby boy who grew to be a tall handsome man. In 1960, she gave birth to a baby girl. Aliza fell pregnant four more times but lost each baby. She recalls that fellow prisoner Germaine Pichon gave birth to a baby boy, who she named Schmel in memory of Samuel. It was found that Aliza and other survivors who had the ovariectomies and later gave birth still had one ovary and half a womb (Shelley 1986, 82). Renée During was exposed to irradiation and underwent three operations destroying the ovary on the right side and survived. Before one of the operations she asked Samuel if she was going to be a guinea pig. He replied, 'I don't think so.' Renée gave birth to a baby girl in 1954. Rosette van Thin, another subject in Block 10, recalls Samuel at a time when 'there were about 20 Jewish women. And this doctor Samuel was going to experiment with one of the women and cut their female organs out. But he never did' (Weinberger 2005, 267).

The experiments in Block 10 in which Jewish doctors were forced to participate had long-lasting and soul-destroying effects on most women survivors. The more fortunate ones only had one ovary removed. We will never know all the facts, but this may have been Samuel's legacy. Jay Lifton argues that Samuel was unprofessional and careless during the operations, particularly in respect to anaesthetics, and that his judgment was clouded due to his poor mental state. He maintains, 'certainly most former prisoners I spoke to, Jewish or otherwise, remembered Samuel as either arrogant or pathetic, or both' (Lifton 2000, 251). Lifton's assessment is very harsh for a number of reasons. First, the testimonies of survivors on whom Samuel operated and who subsequently gave birth after the war demonstrate that Samuel was not following orders. That can be interpreted as an act of resistance. Second, Lifton was and never has been in Samuel's shoes. Elie Wiesel (2006) argues that the actions of Holocaust victims and survivors cannot be judged. Primo Levi refused to blame any Holocaust prisoner for their actions. Daniel Nadav asks,

> Was Samuel really a collaborator, as Lifton claimed? His heroic end places such a conclusion in doubt. Is it possible, however, for those who have never had to face such horror and such awful choices to pass judgment on doctors who found themselves in this predicament? (Nadav 2009, 129)

It is not possible to thoroughly examine Samuel's actions in Auschwitz in the context of his life. His early years, his family and parental influences, and education and religious commitment are not known. What we can assume is that from the time he and Lieselotte entered Monowitz, Samuel's obsession was for his daughter to survive Auschwitz. He had lost his wife and it was natural for him to protect his only child. When he was assigned to the hospital in the factories, it is probable he shared his food and clothing with Lieselotte. It appears that when he worked in Block 10 he worked with the Nazis in the mistaken belief he would save his daughter's life. In addition there is no clear evidence of why and how Samuel was put to death. There are no written orders or witness accounts of what occurred, only rumour and conjecture, and it is doubtful if further research on this matter will reveal a definitive answer. Samuel may have been murdered because he was a Geheimnisträger (a keeper of secrets). Another powerful argument is that Samuel knew if he was caught sabotaging the operations, he would be murdered, and that, having lost the will to live, he took ever-greater risks. Frankl argues that to survive, one had to have a reason to keep going, a reason to live. Samuel's daughter had been his reason to live and when that reason no longer existed, he was prepared to die. At that time, and certainly in Auschwitz, being 62 was considered old and Samuel's mind was possibly clouded. However, there is a vast difference between being slow and befuddled and being a collaborator. Historians, such as Jay Lifton, and others have inferred that Samuel was a collaborator, but I could find no testimony or accusation by a prisoner or Jewish doctor who worked with him that stated he was a conspirator. It is a case for decisions made and actions taken on the basis of the human condition under extreme adversity in Samuel's case the belief that if he co-operated with the SS his daughter's life would be saved.

The story of the two Jewish doctors in Block 10 encapsulates aspects of life and coping skills of people under adversity. On the one hand, there was Brewda, a strong-willed, independent and self-assured individual who, even in the most difficult and harrowing situations managed to cope. Through her commitment to caring and comforting patients, she had a will to live. When she had the opportunity to leave Block 10 and return to Majdanek, her previous camp, she refused out of her concern for the patients. Nevertheless, she was human, fragile and vulnerable as demonstrated by some of her actions. On the other hand, because of the lack of knowledge about Samuels from memoirs or oral testimony we must assume he either collaborated with the SS for reasons unknown, or he had a reason to live and work with the SS to keep his daughter alive. While his daughter was alive he had the will to live. Thus, we assume when he discovered his daughter perished, he lost the will to live, he betrayed the SS and was executed. Both Brewda and Samuel had the status of 'privileged' prisoners, and both displayed similar characteristics of determination, inventiveness and resilience.

The cases of these two doctors attest to the complexities and fragility of survival in Auschwitz. Each doctor was constantly tested, and when in the eyes of the SS they failed the test, they were severely punished: Brewda sent to Block 11; Samuel executed. This demonstrates that the life of Jewish doctors was expendable and that, despite their courage and sacrifices, they were humans driven by personal interests and needs as well as attempting to stay faithful to their professional ethics. Block 10 was unique in the sense that it was a laboratory where goodness and evil can be compared. During human experiments at one end of the operating table was the SS doctor, who abandoned the Hippocratic Oath and the main tenet of 'non nocere', to do no harm, causing harm, suffering and death to innocent people. The Jewish and arguably the non-Jewish prisoner doctors were attempting to uphold their commitment, yet through no fault of their own, failing. The grotesque experiments and vicious cruelty of the SS doctors were surreal to the Jewish doctors. They could neither express professional or personal outrage nor take actions to oppose or halt the SS doctors. They were helpless to stop those atrocities. They could not call upon colleagues or higher authorities to protest. The Jewish doctors in Block 10 and all those who participated in experiments were closely monitored. Under constant threat of punishment or execution, any opposition would be futile. They had no real choice. What is incongruous is that the SS and Jewish doctors came from similar and in some cases the same backgrounds. All doctors received the same medical training with emphasis on the care and welfare of the patient and most had a similar social background coming from middle to upper-class families. Brewda and Dering actually attended the same university and enrolled in the same medical school.

6 Daily Life

The camp had its own ethics, its own idea of right and wrong. It was the ethics of misery, boundless poverty and total humiliation of a human being. Thoughts seized, bodies suffered, souls died or fell into nothingness.

Dr Rosenzweig (1948, 59)

The two critical problems that confronted the SS were the shortage of doctors and outbreaks of epidemics that threatened the existence of Auschwitz as an industrial hub. The problems grew exponentially by the worsening situation on the warfront in the east against Russia and the deteriorating hygienic conditions in the camps. Add to this crisis the refusal of SS doctors and many non-Jewish doctors to treat Jewish patients it forced the Nazis to do the unthinkable and assign Jewish doctors to the Reviers and hospitals.

Before assignment to the hospitals the doctors worked in the labour squads and carried out normal duties treated as ordinary prisoners. Perl (1984) recalled that life in Auschwitz began at four o'clock in the morning, 'when we had to crawl forth from our holes to stand for roll call in the narrow streets separating one block from another.' As privileged prisoners, they received slightly more food and better clothing than the average prisoner and some had a separate room or divided area where they slept. However, many Jewish doctors were privileged in name only, particularly those who were assigned to hospitals and infirmaries and clinics in Birkenau and the labour camps. In those places, they were exposed to every type of infectious disease and subject to beatings and under constant threat of death. Ultimately, most suffered the same fate of the majority of Jewish prisoners, namely death.

The everyday life of the Jewish doctors was routine. With the exception of those working in the research centres, they commenced work in the outpatient clinics or the hospitals and infirmaries between 4 and 7 am, depending on the arrangements and circumstances in each camp. Sick or injured prisoners presented themselves to the clinic where they were examined and either sent back to work after minor treatment or admitted to hospital. In the hospitals, the doctors' commenced with the inspection of the block for cleanliness. They ensured the cleanliness of the block that included collecting the dead from the bunks and moving them in piles outside for collection. The prisoner doctor completed the necessary paperwork recording the name, tattoo number, date, time and cause of death and treatment given. Medical records such as fever charts, blood and urine results and X-rays were included in the documentation. They assessed the patients still alive, and both, the Jewish doctor and patients, awaited the

https://doi.org/10.1515/9783110598216-010

SS doctor in fear. The latter would first consult with and then perhaps take advice from the prisoner doctor as to the health of each prisoner. After inspecting but not touching the prisoner, the SS doctor would make his selection, either allowing the prisoner to remain in hospital, be sent back to work or selecting him or her to be murdered by phenol injection, shot or sent to the gas chambers. After selections the Jewish doctor conducted a roll call (Appell) that, under the threat of severe punishment, had to be accurate. This event could take hours, at times even 12 to 18 hours, especially when the numbers involved over one thousand prisoners and the numbers kept changing because a prisoner died during the count or one of the Muselmänner changed places in the line. After roll call, the Jewish doctor attended to patients, completed medical records and attempted to obtain more medication and medical equipment by any method, usually 'organizing' or stealing.

However, doctors quickly came to realize they were confronting illness and disease on a scale that was far beyond their experience and often skills and means. As Dr Aaron Beijlin described the spread of smallpox:

> Illness touched every person...the number of victims were up to three thousand people...this was a phenomenon which was never before described in medical literature...in our country I knew of only two cases of such illness. (Beijlin 1961)

Working in the hospitals and infirmaries of course exposed the doctors to deadly illnesses that could and did strike many of them down. The mental and emotional toll from exposure to the suffering and pain of the prisoners and the inhumanity and evilness of the perpetrators drove many to suicide. They had no respite from the smells and sights of suffering and death. Conditions in the camp were horrendous. The brick-built blocks were without paving, heating or electric light. They were dirty and infested with rats and other vermin. The floors were dirt and when it rained became muddy. The blocks designed to house up to two hundred people or in previous times one hundred horses held up to one thousand prisoners. The prisoners slept on three tier bunks with up to six prisoners on each level, and in the middle of some of the barracks there was a row of holes to be used as toilets. SS Dr Eduard May, a rat control expert who was sent to inspect Auschwitz, wrote the following in his report to the SS Ahnenerbe (ancestral heritage) institute:

> [On] September 13, 1943, I met with SS-Sturmbannführer Pflaum and the garrison doctor there, SS-Hauptsturmführer Dr Wirths in the Auschwitz garrison administration (SS-Obersturmbannführer Möckel) ... Together with Dr Wirths and Dr Pflaum I visited ... the most rat-infested blocks, barracks, sheds etc., and provided precise guidelines on setting out poison prepared according to instructions ... The intensification of the plague of rats and vermin in this vast camp can be explained by the fact that the camp has grown

at extraordinary speed and that the conditions of that speed have repeatedly limited the hygienic arrangements on the grounds of those of a provisional nature. In addition, located in specific parts of the camps of the Auschwitz complex, in the most primitive of ways, is a downright incredible scum in the shape of Poles, Jews, Gypsies, etc. to whom order is a matter of indifference – in part, whole families, which constitutes a constant source of danger. Finally, it should be taken into consideration that the number of personnel absolutely essential to the sanitary-medical service, doctors, hygienists, etc., and the appropriate auxiliary personnel, is in my opinion decidedly too scanty in relation to the enormous numbers of prisoners who – I repeat – are in part half humans completely indifferent to order. (May 1943)

The lack of drinking water and insufficient food caused malnutrition and starvation:

> Standing, wrapped in a blanket, a child, a little boy. A tiny, shaven head, a face with jutting jaws and a salient superciliary arch. Barefoot, he jumps up and down ceaselessly with a frenzy like that of some barbaric dance. He also waves his arms to keep warm. The blanket slips open. It's a woman. A female skeleton. She is naked. Her ribs and pelvic bones are clearly visible. She pulls the blanket up to her shoulders while continuing to dance. The dance of automaton. A dancing female skeleton. Her feet are small, gaunt, bare in the snow. There are living skeletons that dance. (Delbro 1995, 26)

Lack of food quickly brought prisoners to a state of emaciation and extremely poor health that either killed them or made them vulnerable to serious illness such as typhus and spotted fever. Starvation led them to both madness and death. As Adelsberger recalls,

> Whoever has known true starvation knows that hunger is not merely an automatic animalistic sensation in the stomach, but a nerve-shattering pain, an attack on the whole personality. Hunger makes a person vicious and undermines her character. Many of the things prisoners did, things that rightly seem outrageous and monstrous to the outsider, become understandable and to a certain extent excusable when seen from the perspective of starvation. Worn down like this by hunger and no longer in control of myself, I yearned for, I craved something to eat. And then, when right before my eyes, two non-Jewish Polish aides who had permission to travel started to smear their boots with margarine, starvation made me howl and sob like a child. (Adelsberger 1969, 45)

Olga Lengyel, a Jewish nurse, recalls,

> Our water ration was absurdly minute. Tortured by thirst, we never missed a chance to exchange our meager pittances of bread or margarine for a half pint of water. Better to endure hunger than that hell-fire that was constantly gnawing at our gullets. The water that came through the rusted washroom pipes had an evil smell, a very suspicious color and was hardly fit to drink...This water was better than the rain which stagnated in the puddles; some internees lapped this slop like dogs and died. (Lengyel 1995, 56)

As Beijlin experienced the conditions of deprivation of food:

> The whole time, from morning, we had nothing to eat. Around 11 pm a few cauldrons of green nettle soup and bread (square loafs) were brought in. Six portions were cut out of the loaves. One loaf weighed around 700–800 grams and had sawdust inside. (Beijlin 1961)

The conditions in the camp drove prisoners to the point of madness. To survive they were forced to commit acts against their fellow prisoners that in normal times would be completely foreign to their natural behaviour. Sam Bankhalter spoke of the ruthless drive to survive:

> What I found is that ... human beings in general, we live by circumstances, everybody is able to steal, to kill, to do everything what he ought to do at the proper time. If you have to survive. We all have the instincts. The question is, when does it come into play? And what I saw is, for example, people, they came in with, they're called intelligentsia, people that are very intelligent, doctors, lawyers, uh, philosophers, scientists, you name it. They didn't have a rough life before they came in camp. They didn't survive for very long. They just didn't survive. And the ones that did want to survive, they became the biggest animals that you can ever saw, in order to survive. Now these are people, which of course, had, uh, some background of behaviour, intelligence, and you name it, but it didn't work like that ... these were the ones that would push you, these are the ones they will steal from you, these are ones that will lie in order to survive, so I feel very strongly that circumstances plays a tremendous role, not the way we're brought up, not the way you learn to school, uh, survival, you will do a lot of things which you never thought you will do in order to survive. (Bankhalter 1992)

According to Fejkiel, at first the prisoner behaved with dignity and honesty. As conditions worsened, the lack of food led to hunger and then starvation that created a situation where there were no boundaries, and the people acted like animals. Starving people transformed into people with no willpower or ability to co-operate or act as normal humans. Fejkiel witnessed a father repeatedly stealing food from his feverish son and eating it; on another occasion, he saw a stronger prisoner strangling a neighbour to steal his food (Fejkiel, 1994). Richard van Dam, a medical orderly in Birkenau, recalled that the corruption of human and ethical standards took place rapidly: 'there was constant stealing of blankets and food. Often patients hastened the death of their neighbour so that they could take his portion of bread' (Van Dam 1950). The prisoners were in such a poor state of health in both body and mind that morale deteriorated quickly, and one had to be stern in order to prevent the somewhat stronger patient hastening the death of weaker co-prisoners. The gravity of the fight for survival even extended into the infirmaries:

> There were smarty pants who hung around the rooms in the infirmary in search of dying patients. When such a person saw someone 'at death's door,' he approached him, put his hands on his forehead and then under his head, said a brief prayer, and finally blessed the moribund person with his right hand while retrieving from under that person's head

with his left hand a slice of bread, the existence of which he had verified during his initial inspection. (Langbein 2004, 210)

In the face of physical illnesses, the task of Jewish doctors was nigh impossible. Epidemics and dysentery was the scourge of the camp and seemingly impossible to suppress and eradicate. Typhus, typhoid, spotted fever, diphtheria and malaria swept through the camps in waves while dysentery was a permanent chronic disease. Some doctors may have experienced such circumstances in the ghettos but not on such a large scale. Nyiszli explains why and how dysentery occurred:

> You snatched a person – man, woman or child – from their home and having first robbing them of all their belongings and weakening them during a six-week stay in a crowded ghetto, you then packed them together with hundreds of other people into a cattle truck to be sent off all the way to Auschwitz with the only provisions being one bucket of foul water. Then this person along with thousands of other prisoners, would be put in a barracks where conditions were unfit for a stable. Like everyone else all they had to eat was mouldy (sic) bread, which was in fact a baked mixture of flour and sawdust, synthetic margarine and three decagrams of sausage made from the meat of a mangy horse – all together this amounted to 700 calories a day. The said victim washed all this down with soup made from nettles or swede, without any salt or flour. Within four or five days they had diarrhea. Within three or four weeks the disease would run its course and, regardless of even the tenderest (sic) medical care, our human guinea pig would inevitably die. (Nyiszli 1993, 77)

Once contagious diseases took hold in the camp, spreading from one block to another, the death toll soared. The following table reflects the consequences of a

Table 3: Daily Death Toll by Phenol Injection as a result of Typhus Epidemic.

Date	No. Murdered
Jul-20	150
21	128
22	139
23	140
24	184
25	234
26	99
27	191
28	228
29	116
30	107
31	145
	1861

typhus epidemic in 1942, when over a ten-day period 1,800 Jewish prisoners were murdered by phenol injection in a frantic effort to control the spread of the disease.

The Nazis' strategy to combat epidemics was haphazard and indiscriminate. In the early stages of the outbreak of epidemics a prisoner who had a fever or any sign of contagion would be executed. Nyiszli recalls that Mengele's solution for epidemics was to first quarantine the blocks and isolate the infected prisoners and then, after several days, send them to the gas chambers, shoot or burn them alive. These actions resulted in the extermination of the Czech camp prisoners of three barracks in section C (BIIc).

> On Mengele's order, a strict quarantine was imposed on the prisoners of the barracks where disease symptoms had been identified as well as those of the two neighboring barracks. The quarantine lasted from early morning until evening, when lorries took the inhabitants of all three barracks to the crematorium. Such were the measures Dr Mengele resorted to in an attempt to effectively check the outbreak of an epidemic. (Nyiszli 1993, 70)

The situation became so critical that death blocks were established. Block 20 in the main camp, Block 25 (women's camp) and Block 7 (men's camp) in Birkenau housed typhus patients. Vaisman remembers:

> Block 25 in the Birkenau camp is a block for women condemned to death. The 'selected' are brought there, locked up, guarded carefully by the SS and by personnel of the block, with the blocova at the head, who beats them deprives them of food, refuses them a little water to drink...they waited for the number of the condemned to reach a thousand. They sometimes waited for many days, for the gas chambers could contain a thousand people. (Vaisman 2005, 48)

Two opposing forces were in play by the two cadres of doctors. On the one hand the SS would unhesitatingly condemn sick prisoners to the gas chambers. On the other, the Jewish doctor was committed to protecting prisoners and healing any who could return to work.

> Medicines had to be organized by bribery, or smuggled into the camp...to fight diarrhea, the prisoners ate charcoal from burned bread crusts or pieces of wood. To quench the bleeding, they inserted suppositories made of paper or linen into the anus. They rubbed the main areas infected by scabies with urine, or a salve made of slaked lime and lubricating oil...People went without sleep in order to remove the lice manually at night. Against typhus, the only effective remedy was to apply cold compresses – or to hide the sick. (Czech 1990, 210)

Healing also included mending bodies broken by torturous long days of hard labour. The prisoners were literally worked to death and this was more than evident when the gangs returned back to camp. Broken bones and cuts and bruises were difficult to treat when bandages and medication were almost non-existent. Doctors used paper as bandages and needed every ounce of inventiveness, courage and determination to fight and overcome the obstacles. Dr Rosenzweig was assigned to Block 18F to work with patients with injuries and less serious illnesses such as arthritis, kidney stones, nausea, and anaemia.

> We cured patients mostly with good words, sitting with patients and listening to their complaints. Medication was very limited and scarce. What we got from the pharmacy was quickly used up -codeine calcium. Medication for heart problems we received two tablets a day (very scarce and valuable) and kept for emergencies. We used white clay as antiseptic and as enemas – the latter orally. White clay was also used to paint walls and bunks. (Rosenzweig 1948, 57)

While in the block, Rosenzweig wrote a poem mocking her comprehensive training when all that was available for treatment in the block was white clay.

> *Mam dyplom z Wiednia*
> *Lecz wiedza ma nieodpowiednia*
> *To czegośmy się uczyły, to nie byłO nic*
> *To były kawały, to był głupi witz.*
> *Obóz nam pokazał, gdzie jest mądrość cała:*
> *Jedno jest panaceum: zwie się Glinka biała* (Rosenzweig 1948).

> *I have a degree from Vienna*
> *But my knowledge is inadequate*
> *What we have learned was for nothing*
> *The camp has shown us the wisdom*
> *It was just a hoax, it was for nothing*
> *There is only one panacea: it is called White Clay* [64]

Muselmänner

Professor Jan Obrychi described the Muselmanner as apathetic, drowsy and weakening of the entire life process, particularly the psychic kind. They had bad vision and hearing and their apperception, association, train of thought, and any kind of reaction had slowed down. Thousands of prisoners who had given up hope died a slow agonizing death. They lost the desire to live. The shock of the conditions and brutality and obvious projection of them as sub-human never to leave Auschwitz alive broke many souls and thus the essence of life. Most had lost a loved one or friend. They had been abandoned and they were alone and

---

[64] Translation from Polish to English by Agata Sowinska, Sydney.

isolated. The prisoner separated from a loved one's wife, children, parents – and not knowing their fate suffered what Pauline Boss terms 'ambiguous loss'.[65] The pain of loss and not knowing the fate of their relative became so traumatic that the prisoner could not function as a normal person. As Boss puts it, for people suffering ambiguous loss, 'relational and emotional processes freeze; day-to-day functions and tasks don't get done. Roles and status become confusing. Often people don't know how to act or what to do' (Boss, 2006, 7).

Dr Bruno Bettelheim (1960, 146) contends that the loss of desire to live was a key factor in the majority of deaths in the camps and that prisoners 'simply died of exhaustion, both physical and psychological, due to a loss of desire to live.' He argues further that the majority of the thousands of prisoners died soon after 'deteriorating into a death-like state' (Bettelheim 1960, 146). A person in this condition was called a Muselmänn. As Primo Levi describes:

> [L]ost ones … form the nerve of the camp: they make up the anonymous, constantly renewable and always identical mass of silently marching and overworked nonhumans, they have lost all godly spark, they are so empty that they barely suffer anymore. One hesitates to call them living beings, one hesitates to call their death, of which they are not afraid, death, because they are too tired to grab it …I remember their faceless presence; I could use this familiar image to sum up the entire suffering of our age: a broken man, chin down and crooked shoulders, whose face and eyes show no trace of thinking. (Levi 1989, 29)

The torment of a doctor was witnessing the slow deterioration of the prisoners physically and mentally and a feeling of helplessness. The prisoner needed the skills of a psychiatrist not a general practitioner or a gynaecologist. According to Höss these prisoners accepted the reality that there was no way out. They knew without exception that they were sentenced to death, and that they would stay alive only as long as they could work. The Muselmänner decided not to work, they refused to follow orders, to take care of themselves in regard to sanitary matters, even to eat. Patiently they allowed all the misery, depravation, and torment to happen to them. The hopelessness of escaping the foreseeable end caused them to become totally withdrawn from what was happening in the camp. This mental breakdown accelerated the physical breakdown. They no longer had the will to live. They had become indifferent to everything and even the slightest physical shock caused them to die. Sooner or later death was certain for them (Höss 1996, 142).

---

65 This term is used by Pauline Boss to define such loss as where either a loved one is physically absent but psychologically present or where it is not known whether the person is dead or alive, for example, in the case of a kidnapping, a lost family member, or a relative who is a prisoner of war or hostage. The term is also used where a relative or loved one is physically present but psychologically absent, such as with sufferers of Alzheimer's disease, dementia, brain injury, autism, depression, addiction or other emotional or physical illnesses (Boss, 2006).

Lucie Adelsberger

Dr Lucie Adelsberger worked in Birkenau and survived. She received sufficient food and clothing to stay alive but was affected physically and psychologically. She lived where she worked so she could not escape the spectre of sickness and death even for a few hours. Her memoirs provide an insight into the terrible conditions that prevailed and beg the question of how she survived not only physically, but how she was able to withstand witnessing the complete breakdown of people's bodies and minds. The inability to heal patients and the inescapable observation of the needless and senseless death of hundreds sometimes thousands had their effects. Interestingly, she refers to a copy of Robinson Crusoe that she carried with her everywhere, and which she believed provided her with some strategies to survive Auschwitz. Unfortunately, she does not elaborate, but we can assume that Crusoe's inventiveness, hope and coping skills gave her inspiration.

Lucie Adelsberger was born in Nuremberg on 12 April 1895. Her father, Isidor Adelsberger, was a wine merchant. Her mother, Rosa Lehmann, was a stay-at-home mother. She had a younger brother and sister. When Isidor died, the family continued to live in Nuremberg. Lucie attended the local Städtische Töchterschule (public girls' school) for nine years and spent four years at the Privat-Real-Gymnasium Dr Uhlemayr (a private high school). In 1919 she completed her medical degree from the University of Erlangen-Nuremberg; the following year she commenced worked as a medical assistant at the Cnopf'sche Kinderklinik in the neo-natal ward. In 1921 she left for Berlin and worked in the paediatric and internal medicine department of the municipal hospital in Berlin-Friedrichshain, where she remained for twenty years specializing in immunology and allergies.

Lucie was subject to antisemitism from an early age. This–interfered with her studies and career. After graduation Adelsberger suffered similar abuse and criticism, as did most Jewish doctors, for monopolising medicine in Germany. After Hitler's rise to power, she along with her colleagues found it difficult, then impossible, to work in the medical profession. Instead they were only able to work as jüdische Krankenbehandler, Jewish caretakers of the sick rather than doctors. Adelsberger's reputation in the field of bacteriology prompted Harvard University to offer her tenure in their medical faculty during a trip she made to the United States in 1933. Adelsberger rejected the offer and returned home to look after her mother, who could not obtain a visa for the United States. Her mother was the focus of her life. As life for the Jews became more menacing, many families were concerned for the wellbeing of their elderly parents. Adelsberger too worried about how to protect her mother from suffering at the hands of the Nazis:

Many people did manage to give their parents some liberating sedative. I found comfort in the thought at first, but then, when the roundups increased and the time came ever nearer, I began to waiver...was I, who had spent her whole life struggling to save each and every human life, was I supposed to kill my mother, the person so dear to me in all the world? May a person who trusts in a higher power ever deliberately end a life, be it her or that of another? I couldn't do it. (Adelsberger 1969, 12)

To Lucie's relief her mother died shortly before she was deported to Auschwitz from Berlin on 17 May 1943. Adelsberger was initially assigned to the gypsy camp and then to Birkenau when the gypsies were liquidated in July 1944. Her account of her experiences in Auschwitz as a prisoner and doctor describe in detail the conditions, suffering and, most importantly, the life of an ordinary Jewish doctor as opposed to that of the more privileged prisoner doctor in the experimental sectors. She worked at the outpatient clinic for almost two years and commenced work at four in the morning. The conditions in the gypsy camp were horrible; the blocks were no more than unconverted horse stables.

It had no windows, and the scant light it did admit entered through a narrow ribbon of glass that ran beneath the roof rafters. The wind blew with all its fury through the broad crevices in the wooden walls; cold and heat penetrated unobstructed, and the rain streamed through the holes and cracks in the inadequately tarred roof, soaking the dirt floor as well as the patients' bunks. Both longitudinal walls of the block were lined with as many 'beds' as could be crammed in, three-tiered wooden bunks with boards that didn't fit and constantly shifted around in every direction. (Adelsberger 1969, 36)

Her living conditions were no better than those of the patients.

Our 'beds', two straw sacks for three people on the lowest level of a three-tiered bunk reserved for patients; in addition she gave us two filthy blankets stickily (sic) encrusted with spittle and excrement. The whole arrangement wasn't very inviting, particularly the announcement of our neighbours that, not two hours before, the previous inhabitants, typhus patients, had died just in time to make room for us. Disinfection? Not as a rule! You're going to get it, anyway. (Adelsberger 1969, 37)

Adelsberger worked in conditions that were totally inadequate. Along the length of the block were two wooden tables on which the doctors sat to write or update medical reports and fever charts. The was also a stove:

[which] was the focal point of every activity; people climbed over it with their dirty belongings whenever they wanted to get from one side to the other. Injections were given and abscesses lanced ...we ate there, 'cooked' there, washed there with the little water we had – contaminated, filthy brown water that stained everything yellow because of its iron content ...frequently enough, we even slept on top of this stove. (Adelsberger 1969, 35)

Living with the patients Lucie could never escape the utter desolation and dejection.

Where the sickly who no longer had the strength to sit up or crawl out of bed to attend to their business were berthed, was a mire of faeces – and urine-drenched blankets. The dying writhed among the dead, emitting a dull, extended moan that sounded like the cry of an animal perishing in the forest primeval. (Adelsberger 1969, 38)

One of her most dreaded responsibilities was counting patients at roll call. Everything had to reconcile, with the threat of whipping, twenty-five strokes of the oxtail, if the records were inaccurate. The task of ensuring accurate records of the number of patients was made harder with death occurring by the minute in some cases. On most occasions people had died by the time they had finished counting so they had to recount. She recalls that once,

I had made five head counts, but the total never came out right. One patient was always missing, and there was never an answer when her number was called. Maybe she had died and her body been tossed on the hearse before she could be counted or deleted from the list. (Adelsberger 1969, 39)

Adelsberger confesses she could not have endured the whipping 'only strong men lived through that' (Adelsberger 1969, 39). The time spent counting prisoners meant less time treating patients. Difficulties were compounded by the lack of medicine and supplies. She recollects the scant necessities they had at hand and introducing the use and dependency on the same clay Rosenzweig referred to, a white powder that became the cure-all for almost every complaint:

The only thing we did have in any quantity was bolus alba,[66] not in boxes or bags but by the sackful. Bolus, this white powder, was our panacea; it was given internally for diarrhoea, dabbed on mucous membranes in cases of stomatitis and sprinkled over inflammations of the skin. (Adelsberger 1969, 40)

Frequently doctors had nothing to offer patients but emotional support.

The only thing the doctors could do for their patients emaciated, skeletal, or swollen with oedema of starvation and wallowing in feverish deliriums as they were, was to comfort and encourage them. It didn't make them any better: they still died like flies. (Adelsberger 1969, 40)

On 18 January 1945 Adelsberger went on the infamous death march to Ravensbrück that took nine days. Conditions there were even worse than in Auschwitz:

---

[66] Latin for any mass of medicinal material, usually in pill form but capable of being powdered by crushing. The aim of the medicine manufactured from herbs was to help the organism to heal itself thereby allowing the body, soul and spirit to recover.

> We lay for a full day in the dirty snow piled high against the walls of the camp avenue, still without food or drink…toward evening eight thousand people were herded into a machine shed, where a bowl of camp soup and a few potatoes awaited those skilled in pushing and shoving their way to the front. (Adelsberger 1969, 125)

Adelsberger's life in Auschwitz, the Death March and her internment in Ravensbrück tell a story of survival under the most extreme conditions. For almost two years terror, brutality, atrocious sanitary conditions, sickness and death were her constant companions. Neither could she escape the smell of burning human flesh and the screams and crying of those taken to the gas chambers and fire pits. Lucy Adelsberger's story provides a window into the human condition under adversity in relation to how circumstances change behaviour. In the beginning she told of her love and devotion to her mother and her willingness to sacrifice her career to return home to care for her mother. Then with the advancement of the Nazis she could not bring herself to kill her invalid mother as so many of other children did to save their parents from the enemy. Yet once in Auschwitz, when she was aborting foetuses, killing new-born babies and unwillingly participate in selections that decided which patient would live or die and waking up covered in excrement or next to a person who had died during the night she changed. Adelsberger's actions were typical of the behaviour of a human being under extreme adversity and as a consequence of the human condition. During the Death March when a young girl needed her help to walk and Lucie did not have the strength to carry both of them, she released the girls grip knowing she would be shot or beaten to death. Her decisions were made out of determination to live. Although Lucie had high standards of personal values, medical ethics, morality and religious faith her will to live was paramount. I have said and quoted Primo Levi that no Holocaust victim or survivor can be judged for their actions.

After World War II Dr Lucie Adelsberger migrated to the United States and worked at the Montefiore Hospital and Medical Center in New York City as an immunologist. She died in 1971 at the age of 76.

7 Ethical Dilemmas. Choiceless Choices and the Human Condition

It is a grey zone, with ill-defined outlines, which both separate and join the two camps of masters and servants. It possesses an incredibly complicated internal structure, and contains within itself enough to confuse our need to judge.

Primo Levi (1989)

Jewish doctors in Auschwitz often made decisions that caused or contributed to the death of a prisoner or some prisoners. Under everyday normal conditions judgments of what is right or wrong are determined by many factors such as family guidance, religious beliefs, moral standards, professional ethics, education, cultural impact and so on. Due to the loss of freedom and choice in Auschwitz they lacked the opportunity to benefit from these valuable resources. They were isolated and alone.

The common theory today is the Jewish doctors mainly faced ethical dilemmas when treating and inter-acting with patients. Based on the conditions, inhumanity and suffering in the camp which I have already addressed linked to the overwhelming number of patients, complexity of the diseases and illnesses and finally the demands of the Nazis it is inconceivable that the Jewish doctor was only confronted by ethical dilemmas. In addition to his or her role as a doctor they were humans with the same innate drive to survive. As Jews they were under a sentence of death that was imminent. Thus the decisions made were influenced and driven by the human condition and by what Lawrence Langer refers to as 'choiceless choices'. In Auschwitz where survival was a powerful and all-consuming goal, the reasons for certain behaviours were uncomplicated. Under circumstances when death was pending the will to live governed decisions and actions. A prisoner under a death sentence with the exception of the extraordinary person would commit any offence and abandon personal values and morality, codes of ethics and religious tenets in order to survive. Prisoners quickly learned on entering the camp they were alone. According to Levi:

> One entered hoping at least for the solidarity of one's companions in misfortune, but the hoped-for allies, except in special cases, were not there; there were instead a thousand sealed-off monads, and in between them a desperate hidden and continuous struggle. This brusque revelation, which became manifest from the very first hours of imprisonment, often in the form of concentric aggression on the part of those in whom one hoped to find future allies, was so harsh as to cause the immediate collapse of one's capacity to resist. (Levi 1989, 23)

Levi (1989) introduces the concept of the 'grey zone', those prisoners he calls functionaries, the privileged and 'Prominente', who were somewhere between

https://doi.org/10.1515/9783110598216-011

the perpetrators and victims. Their numbers were limited but their power and influence was considerable and their actions often meant the difference between the life and death of the prisoners.

> Without regard to ability and merit, power is generously granted to those willing to pay homage to hierarchic authority, thus attaining an otherwise unattainable social elevation. (Levi 1989, 32)

Levi writes that it was common for Kapos, Lagerältesten, Blockältesten and other designated prisoners to be ruthless and cruel, sometimes killing fellow Jews, in carrying out their orders. They would rationalize that their motives were to stay alive and their brutality was to keep their status that in turn enabled them to stay alive. The result, according to Levi, were:

> The 'saved' of the Lager were not the best, these predestined to do good; the bearers of a message... Preferably the worst survived, the selfish, the violent, the insensitive, the collaborators of the 'grey zones,' the spies. It was not a certain rule (there were none, nor are there certain rules in human matters), but it was, nevertheless, a rule... The worst survived – that is, the fittest; the best all died. (Levi 1989, 62)

Levi judges the 'privileged' prisoners. Elie Wiesel and Jean Améry are amongst many survivors who insist those who haven't walked in the prisoners' shoes can't make judgment. As a survivor of Auschwitz Levi is qualified to make judgment but admits he could be accused of bias in his assessment. While he concentrates on the actions of Kapos and some categories of prisoners as well as members of the Ghetto Judenrat Councils, Levi singles out Jewish doctors as the largest group of survivors in the 'grey zone'. Granted, the doctors were human beings and not infallible as they each demonstrated. But were they violent, selfish, and insensitive? Were they collaborators? If they were 'privileged' prisoners, why did the likes of Vaisman, Perl, Adelsberger, Wolken and Grunwald live and work in Birkenau, the worst camp in the Nazi-occupied territory and arguably the cruellest and most murderous place in history? Did the doctors have any guidelines when making choices?

Jewish doctors faced dilemmas that challenged them in every aspect of their life and work in Auschwitz. I would contend that within the framework of their professional codes, personal values and morality, they were driven by the will to live, the threat of death or beatings and the care and well-being of their patients, and I am not sure in what order these factors line up. The question of ethics, morality and religion may have been present in the initial instances of Jewish doctors' active involvement in selections, human experiments and even killing fellow prisoners but my thesis is that as time went on and involvement in terrible activities increased, the emotional and ethical impact on the Jewish doctor diminished. The doctors became detached from the suffering and death and dehumanized to such an extent that their actions and responses became robotic. How could Perl and Adelsberger and many other Jewish doctors continue time and time again to abort foetus and kill new born babies or chose which patient would live and who would die when handing out medication?

Were the choices confronting Perl, Adelsberger and Brewda dilemmas? Perl made it her mission to save the lives of pregnant prisoners. This gave her life meaning. Did aborting a foetus or killing a newborn to save the life of the mother present her with a dilemma? According to her memoirs she had no choice. She was committed to save the life of the mother. The alternative was to allow the pregnancy to come to full term and both mother and child would be executed. Adelsberger faced the same challenge and met it with similar conviction. It could be said the doctors established a personal 'Auschwitz' code of ethics and morals in response to this situation. They were doing the lesser of two evils. Deciding which patient would receive the one tablet available or choosing the criteria which would determine which prisoner was selected for execution will have been made according to each doctor's code that justified or allowed him or her to rationalize the decision. Dutch Jewish doctor Eli Cohen initially felt that he faced a dilemma when told to quiet disruptive patients or he and the whole block would be exterminated. But, seeing no alternative way to do it, he chose to kill a noisy patient using insulin to save his own life and those of the block patients:

> We had a large supply of insulin – I don't know how we got hold of it... 200 units of insulin. And from then on it was quiet in our block. On that occasion I... yes, I infringed the ethical rule that one is a doctor not to murder people, but to try to keep them alive, to try to cure them, help them. And... it's always the first step that counts. For a few weeks later, it happened again. But by that time I had far fewer moral scruples about going upstairs again and saying to Valentin, 'Same old thing. We'll have to do it again. And we did too, and that man died as well. (Cohen 1973, 88)

After that first decision, Cohen faced no further sense of dilemma – he would sacrifice individual patients to save the lives of many.

Albert Haas, was standing in line during a selection. He realized that according to the count he would be chosen for the gas so he manhandled the prisoner next to him to exchange places and save his own life. The prisoner was a Muselmänn, so emaciated and extremely weak so pushing him was effortless. He justified his decision on the basis the prisoner was soon going to die. In other words, he 'selected' the prisoner to die. He cannot have considered it a dilemma because in a matter of seconds he made the decision to save his own life. Nothing in his memoirs indicates he gave his actions much thought other than the imminent danger to his own life. Haas under the circumstances was acting as a normal person under the circumstances not as a doctor. Irrespective there is no right or wrong. In such cases ethics and morality are nebulous. The Jewish doctors in their memoirs did not address the subject of dilemmas nor did they refer to religion or the Hippocratic oath when death was imminent. Doctors such as Cohen, Perl and Adelsberger did question their actions in causing the death of fellow prisoners but it did not stop them. Being instrumental in taking one prisoner's life meant saving another. Was Primo Levi harsh in making the judgement that only the worst kind of prisoner survived? Did he omit something from his memoirs?

There is only one piece of evidence to suggest that a Jewish doctor refused to follow SS orders: Brewda's refusal to operate on victims of sterilization experiments. She was eventually sentenced to Block 11 and lost her privileged status. The threat of beatings and death motivated the Jewish doctor to follow orders. As Dvorjetski states, other doctors were unable to face the responsibility of the difficult decisions that confronted them and chose to hide their profession and even die rather than participate in selections or human experiments:

> They [Jewish prisoner doctors] have faced in some of the camps, many terrific problems, because the Nazi doctors and SS men, wanted to use them, by threatening and tortures [sic], as instruments to carry on Nazi evil devices, and had forced upon them operations against their conscience … I know quite a number of events when Jewish doctors had hidden their profession from the Germans, because they feared they could not stand the proof [sic], and had chosen to work hard works than to be a doctor in the camp … a lot of cases are known to me when Jewish doctors were beaten to death or murdered by Nazi doctors, or by SS men, because they did not want to carry on their bloody orders; I know many cases of seldom occurrence of Jewish doctors who had committed suicide in concentration camps, because they could not continue such a low life. (Dvorjetski 1952, 4)

It will never be known how many doctors who entered the camp committed suicide or hid their profession.

Is there a distinction between one type of killing and another? The Jewish doctor killed many Jewish prisoners. Albeit unwillingly, the Jewish doctor actively participated in the killing of fellow prisoners or caused the death of a prisoner through omission by deciding not to give necessary medicine to another. There is passive participation in killing even when the most humane decision regarding patients in a critical state of health, living in such reprehensible conditions and with no chance of survival would be to assist them to die.

After the Holocaust some Jewish doctors, such as Perl, Cohen and Adelsberger expressed guilt and shame for their actions in Auschwitz. Cohen felt guilt for having killed prisoners. Perl and Adelsberger expressed guilt and pain for aborting foetuses and killing newborn babies. Brewda felt guilt for not being able to save her patients from pain and eventual death. Taking part in selections troubled Micheels. Vaisman was disturbed by what she witnessed in the camp admitting she was helpless and was unable to warn new arrivals of their fate. Albert Haas, a prisoner of several concentration camps including Auschwitz stated 'even today, I still question decisions I made.' He felt:

> It is natural that the Jewish doctors would feel guilty and ashamed for their involvement in the death of fellow prisoners and anger towards the SS for creating dilemmas. Surely the blame rests not with those forced to make such choices, but with those responsible for creating the circumstances in which such choices must be made. (Haas 1984, xi)

Perhaps what Primo Levi is so judgemental about in regard to Jewish prisoner doctors is that he thought they lacked empathy. We associate care with empathy and concern, and both are attributes we like doctors to show. What motivated the Jewish doctors in their role as healers – empathy or concern? Obviously, they felt both to some extent but there is an important distinction between the two. Empathy is putting oneself in another's shoes; it is sharing the feelings of others, especially feelings of sorrow and anguish. Concern is worrying about the welfare of another, wanting to care for another. One can have concern for another without having empathy. Prinz (2011) suggests that concern 'often seems to involve an element of moral anger.' This definition resonates with what we know of the doctors who survived. The moral anger throughout the survivors' memoirs is tangible. Vaisman, Perl, Adelsberger, Micheels and Brewda all express deep contempt and hatred for the Nazis and Nazi doctors, particularly Mengele and Clauwitz.

Doctors had concern for prisoners coming into contact with infected patients. They were concerned for the pain and suffering of prisoners who were beaten and tortured. Feelings of empathy allowed the doctor to relate too deeply to the mental and physical health of the prisoner, and adversely affected the doctor's emotional state and practical capacity to work as a healer. On the other hand concern for the prisoners' welfare inspired the doctor to act. Empathy makes one think and feel. Concern encourages one to act. In almost every case the Jewish doctor acted. In reality they did not have the time to be empathic. How could one feel empathy for thousands of emaciated patients? In most instances the doctor could continue to work under those conditions only if they could detach and distance themselves from the misery and suffering.

In Camus' *The Plague*, Dr Rieux battles with the realization that he is helpless to prevent death from the plague and that he needs to maintain distance from the patient so that his feelings do not prevent him from trying to make impossible decisions. The alternative is to go insane. Camus succinctly describes the true position of the Jewish doctors that they were unable to portray in their memoirs:

His sensibility was getting out of hand. Held back most of the time, hardened and dried out, it would occasionally collapse and abandon him to feelings he could no longer control. His only defence was to resort to hardening himself and tightening the knot that had formed in him. He knew full well that this was the correct way to proceed. For the rest he had few illusions and tiredness took away even those that he still had. He knew that for a period of time, the end of which he could not see, his role was no longer that of a healer; it was that of a diagnostician. Discovering, seeing, describing, noting and then condemning – that was his task. (Camus 2009, 149)

Although the doctor was concerned, moral distancing became a mechanism that enabled him to cope. According to Camus (2009), certain jobs, sometimes of great social value (and, in the case of the Jewish prisoner doctor, of great humane value) might be psychologically too demanding if those doing them did not to some extent work with a deadened imagination or with simple categories limiting their sense of responsibility. They describe feelings of despair and helplessness in their attempts to care for patients, but their participation in selections generated far deeper, more personal feelings of guilt, fear, shame, terror, panic and disbelief. Cohen recalls that every two weeks the SS doctor would visit his block,

Again I told Dr Klein the men's names, and again he handed the charts to the SS man... And the Germans never said these people were going to their death. The Germans always had such fine names for things like that. In this case it was 'SB' – Sonderbehandlung – special treatment. And special treatment meant gas. And that's the way people went who'd lain longer in that room. (Cohen 1973, 91)

On seeing another load of people go to the gas chambers, Cohen recalls, 'suddenly I began to weep. I can still see it. We had a small screened-off corner belonging to the room superior, where we had our meals, being the "leaders" of that room. "But it's so inhuman," I said. "You just can't do a thing like that"' (Cohen 1973, 90).

Selections

Selections were the bane of every Jewish doctor who worked in the hospital system. Although selections have been referred to above the subject needs more attention for the doctors' participation in such a process represented in many cases the death not only of a Jew but the death of the soul of the doctor as a human being and as a healer. In most cases the Nazi doctor did little more than tell the prisoner doctor how many prisoners were required. Lifton writes of a Jewish doctor who admitted that the practice of selections haunted him more than anything else. Patients who were very weak and showed no improvement after days of hospitalization would sooner or later be recognized as unable to work and 'we were unable to help. So they went off ...to the gas chambers – controlled (selected) by the SS doctors. And we would have to decide who he (the SS doctor) would see' (Lifton 2000, 221). Jewish doctors had no alternative but to co-operate. They knew that left to their own devices, the Nazi doctors would select any prisoner irrespective of fitness or health. Thus healthy prisoners or even orderlies or nurses could be selected merely to make up the numbers. Selections in the main took place under two circumstances; in the hospital wards as shown in Fig. 18 and at roll call as illustrated in Fig. 19. The Jewish doctor was intimately involved in the selections in the hospital and infirmaries but played no part in roll call selections.

By co-operating in selections, Jewish doctors could select patients who would not survive another hour or day and thus prolong healthy prisoners' chance at life even if it was only for a short period. This was considered a 'good' selection. A prisoner doctor told how Dr Fritz Klein kept demanding more information about sick patients in order to meet certain quotas for the gas chambers. He confessed:

> It's not honest in life to ask from a man such things. Maybe you have to be a holy man to say no. I'm not optimistic about my own behaviour, you see. And still I am not a bad man. Really not! But life asks me, You or me? And I say, Me!. (Lifton 2000, 221)

Prisoner doctors were usually told in advance of an impending selection. This information could come from various sources including the Schreibstube,

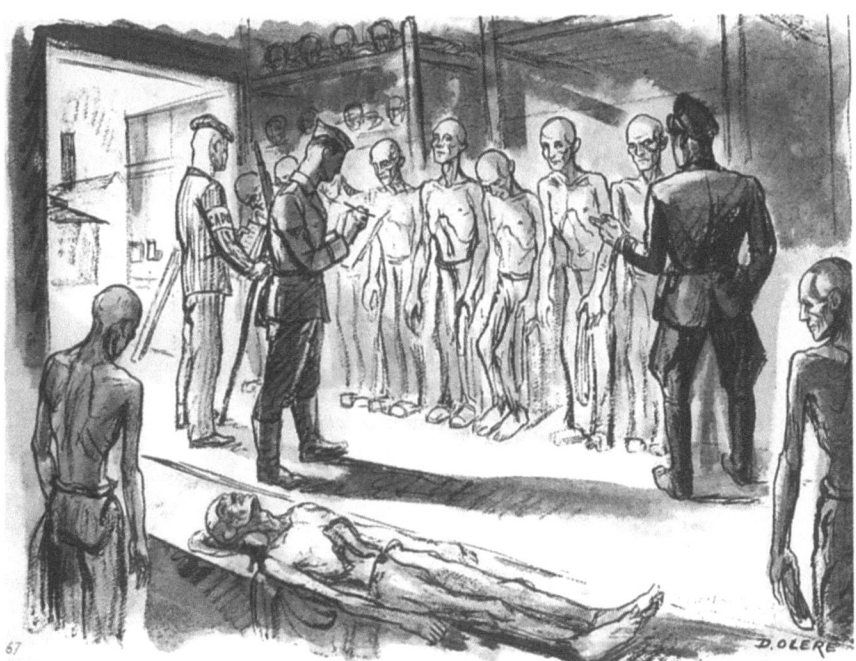

Fig. 18: Selection taking place in a hospital ward. David Olère (1945).

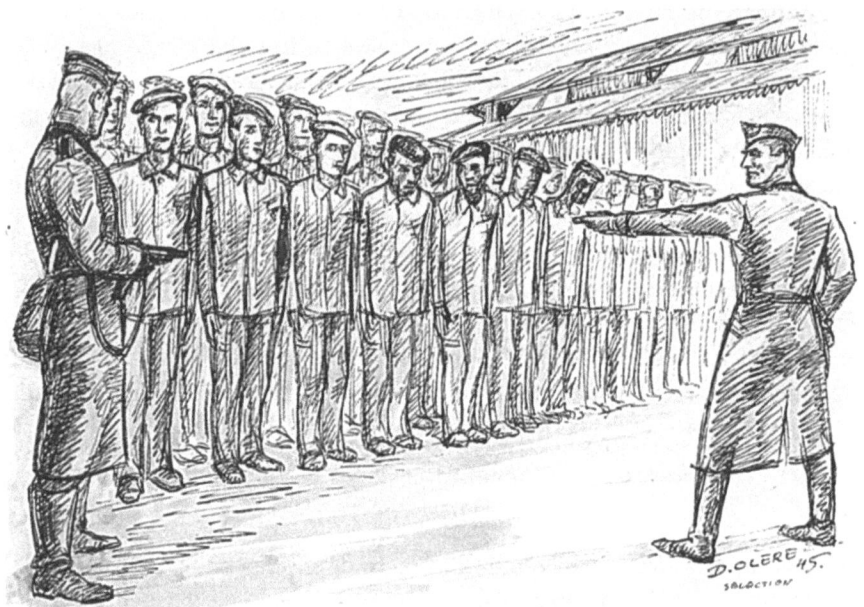

Fig. 19: Selection taking place during roll call. David Olère (ca 1989).

friendly Kapos and even SS guards. This gave the doctors the opportunity to hide patients, to prepare patients for selections by ensuring they appeared healthy (pinching the face of the prisoner to bringing colour to the cheeks), releasing certain prisoners back to their blocks and re-admitting them after the selection, falsifying records, and by saving the life of healthy prisoners by concentrating only on those who were hopeless cases, close to death's door.

Rosenzweig reported the following conversation between himself and the Polish doctor Laniewska, who prepped him on an impending selection:

Laniewska:	You must come as early as 5 am to prepare the block for the selection.
Rosenzweig:	What do I have to do?
Laniewska:	The patient's fever charts that have been on the Block for longer than two weeks must be hidden. The more severe cases of patients who look bad we will hide in the washroom... you cannot give as diagnosis those with bodily pain because these go straight to the ovens. Come at 5 am then we will discuss everything. The selections will take place between 7 and 8 am. We will put the sick in the washrooms.
Rosenzweig:	You mean the ones that look bad and the ones you keep here as 'children'?
Laniewska:	Yes. We will take the keys to the washroom with us.
Rosenzweig:	So they are not going to look in the washroom?
Laniewska:	Usually they don't look – they believe us – but if they look we will answer with our lives – tough – we're in the camps (Rosenzweig 1948, 59).

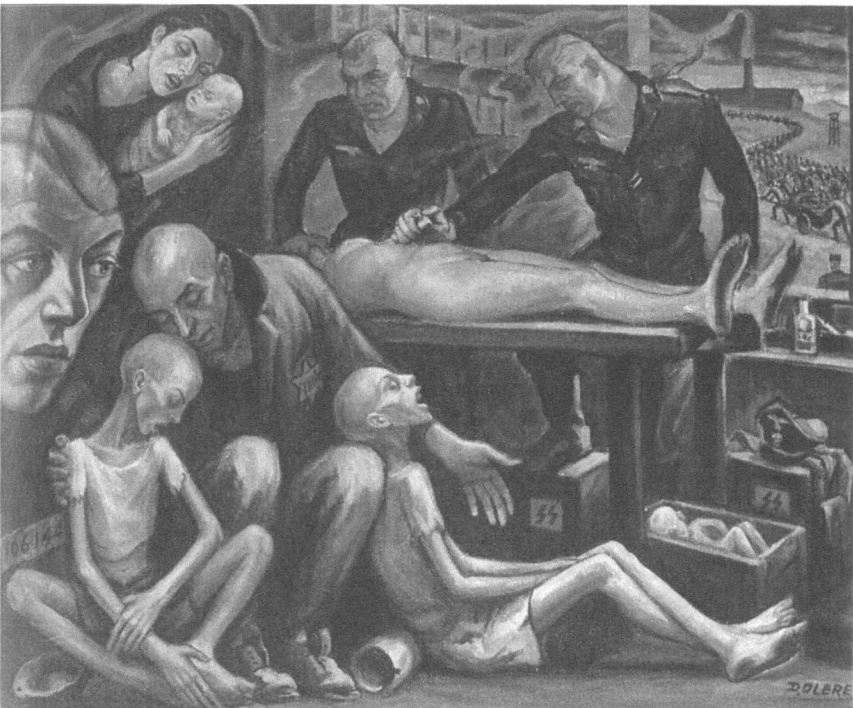

Fig. 20: Death by Phenol Injection after Selection. Olere (1989).

The unendurable scene in Fig. 20 is a response to D.H. Lawrence's question of what is evil? / There is only one evil, to deny life (Lawrence 2008, 29). Micheels recalls a similar approach under his watch but also expresses his emotional response to the situation:

> We had some selections on our wards ...we managed to conceal case records and send those patients with little chance of passing the selection to the bathroom or other hiding places. In this way, even if we could not do very much, they perhaps had a chance of survival, or at least die a natural death. These selections were both infuriating and terrifying. I just could not understand how a doctor with a mere glance could dispose of a human life he had vowed to protect. (Micheels 1989, 87)

Relationship with SS and Non-Jewish prisoner doctors

The attitude of the Nazi doctor towards the Jewish doctor swung between respect and denigration, the latter often leading to brutality. The treatment of Jewish doctors was dependent on their role and status. Those working in the infirmaries and hospitals were often treated no better than the average prisoner. The SS refused to recognize them, saying 'Ein jüdischer Arzt ist kein Artz, sondern ein Abtreiber und Giftmischer.' – a Jewish doctor is not a doctor, but an abortionist and poisoner. Unfortunately the relationship between the Jewish and Polish doctors was fragile and complex. The number of Polish doctors was far greater than that of Jewish doctors. According to Dering, in one of the hospitals in Auschwitz there were approximately 60 doctors of various nationalities of which approximately ten to twelve were Jewish. The latter held senior positions and were recognized and accepted as doctors by the Nazis. The change in policy assigning Jewish doctors to hospitals threatened the status of the non-Jewish doctors. Primo Levi recalls the reception senior prisoners, mainly Polish 'prominents', gave to new prisoners:

> The collision with the concentrationary [sic] reality coincides with the unforeseen and uncomprehended [sic] aggression on the part of a new and strange enemy, the functionary-prisoner, who instead of taking you by the hand, reassuring you, teaching you the way, throws himself at you, screaming in a language you do not understand, and strikes you in the face. (Levi 1989, 30)

He could easily have been talking about the response of established prisoner doctors to the newly arrived Jewish doctor colleagues. Lifton gives the following analysis:

> Long standing Polish antisemitism loomed especially large ... Polish doctors and even worse prisoner orderlies, who really abuse [d] Jews ... in a way that caused people to suffer and to die ... some Poles could make common cause with the authorities in being ... so anti-Semitic they didn't care about the Jews being gassed or [fatal] injections because they had the feeling they were some kind of superior being. (Lifton 2000, 240)

Beatings of Jewish doctors by Polish doctors were common, 'for the Polish or the others to strike a Jew it was no problem' (Lifton 2000, 240). Obviously, as was the case prior to the war, the Jews could not escape humiliation and abuse even in a prison. Hatred followed them everywhere. Beijlin recalls his experience with a prisoner Polish doctor, Dr Zenkeller:

> Every day at dawn Zenkeller already was up and came to inspect both the infirmary and patient's block. One time he met me when I was scrubbing the floors. He didn't like my work and kicked me very hard ... another occasion he asked me for an opinion of the health of a German Kapo. I replied that in my opinion the Kapo was suffering from pleuritis [emphysema]. Zenkeller didn't like my prognosis and called me names – filthy Jew, Talmud lover, only a Talmud lover could come up with such a diagnosis. After he left I took a syringe and drew pus from the lung and being stupid I went to Zenkeller's to show him the pus. Zenkeller saw the syringe telling me to get rid of it and then hit me in the head. I lost consciousness

and when I woke Zenkeller threatened me: 'you will never get out of here … you will end your days here … I give you my word … ask the other prisoners … they know I always keep my word'. He kicked me one more time. (Beijlin 1961)

Dering, a Polish doctor, and fellow university student of Brewda, treated her with contempt in Auschwitz, and was dismissive of her protestations over his unethical behaviour and medical practices in performing cruel and meaningless operations. Brewda describes an incident with Dering:

> During the course of that afternoon ten girls were operated on. These girls were brought over one by one from Block 10. When the girls with irradiation burns were brought in I said to Dr Dering, 'Leave them alone. They are suffering enough already from the burns.' He replied, 'Shut up. I have my orders'. (Minney 1996, 130)

He threatened to report her to the Nazi authorities. In the defamation case in London, Dering was questioned about his dealings with Jewish doctors and Jewish patients. He refused to accept the accusation he was antisemitic, insisting that he worked with the SS to save his own life. Although there were incidences where a Polish doctor was caring and helpful, they were often considered as much an enemy as the Nazis and not to be trusted.

The life of the Jewish doctor did not only involve confronting the conditions of the camp and meeting the demands of the SS and the needs of the prisoners. They were also fighting their own personal demons in relation to defiling religious beliefs, personal values, and professional ethics. Assigned as a doctor to the hospitals, infirmaries and experimental blocks classified them as privileged prisoners. However, status and privilege had its dark side in being made to participate in selections, human experiments and executions.

Part IV: **Survival**

You want to live, at any cost. You want to live because you are alive, because the whole world is alive. There is nothing but life. Zalman Lewental (Grief 2005, 19)

In common usage, the meaning of the word survival has been polarized. In one sense, survival is used in an exaggerated way. People use the expression to describe any situation that places the slightest burden on their lifestyle or wellbeing. When taxes rise or health costs increase the most common reaction is, 'How are we going to survive?' Then there is the person who lies in bed in the foetal position fearful of how survival is possible when they have received a redundancy notice. People often speak of surviving when they really mean they are just getting through life. Lifton may be correct when he stated that man is viewed 'as a perpetual survivor ... of "holocausts" large and small, personal and collective, that define much of existence' (Lifton 2000, 12). Likening normal daily troubles and challenges to minor 'holocausts' may sound extreme nevertheless in western culture today in which life seemingly depends on instant gratification and the self, any deprivation or sacrifice can raise the question of survival more as a threat to one's standard of living than to real suffering or death of another. In another sense, it has been minimized. Globalization and technology bring graphic live coverage of death and destruction into our living rooms on a daily basis. Yet survivors of major catastrophes such as earthquakes, floods, fires and typhoons are soon forgotten. In the process of losing families and possessions they receive brief attention and frequently insufficient assistance and relief from governments and charities. While many millions will die from starvation, disease, inhumanity, war, terrorism and captivity, others will ultimately survive in the true sense of the word and rebuild their lives.

The context in which I have studied survival is where ordinary people, who suddenly find themselves under conditions of extreme adversity and where life is threatened, survive. Despite these extremities the survivor refuses to recognize or submit to the threat of extinction and, although broken in spirit and body, lives on. It raises the question of how do some people rise above and overcome adversity? Under normal conditions of daily life that are mostly predictable and of manageable stress we call upon our usual resources to address issues. But how does one comprehend and confront a place such as Auschwitz in which morality was non-existent replaced by such unimaginable evilness and depravity that resulted in the extermination of over one million Jews? Everything had been taken, identity, appearance, health, dignity, self-esteem, possessions, friends and most precious, family. And then hope disappeared. Replaced by a number, shame, loneliness, ill health, helplessness, despair, hopelessness and finally death. Nevertheless a few survived. Why and how?

https://doi.org/10.1515/9783110598216-012

Dreams used to come in the brutal nights
Dreams crowding and violent
Dreamt with body and soul,
Of going home, of eating, of telling our story.
Until quickly and quietly, came
The dawn reveille:
Wstawàch
And the heart cracked in the breast (Levi 1995, xi)

In extremity, the bare possibility of survival is not enough. There must also be a move beyond despair and self-pity to that fierce determination which survivors call upon in order to pull through. To keep a living soul in a living body he or she must rise above the conditions and the inhumanity, and resist the temptation to take what could be said is 'the easy road' and succumbs to a swift or early death (Des Pres 1976, 7).

The story of the survival of Jewish doctors in Auschwitz presents a unique and never before researched case study under the most horrific and inhumane conditions. It presents us with a microcosm of survival under adversity. When I use the term adversity or extremity I mean a situation where there was no escape and there were only victims and perpetrators. There were no rescuers and thus no protection from the first blow that Améry argued caused the victim to lose 'trust in the world' adding, 'If no help can be expected, this physical overwhelming by the other becomes an existential consummation of destruction altogether (Améry 1986, 28)'.

The Nazis had created an environment that destroyed the prisoner in body and mind. The process of extermination was well planned, and coldly and calmly executed. On learning of the conditions under which most Jewish doctors lived and worked without respite, I wondered if in some way the prisoners who had an early death were not the fortunate ones. My research suggests that the Jewish doctor who survived, including those who were within reach of but tragically denied freedom, died a thousand deaths. They were both witnesses to and victims of a level cruelty and inhumanity so extreme that Eli Wiesel and Primo Levi felt it required a new language to describe it adequately. As Dante Alighieri wrote, 'grief so deep the tongue must wag in vain; the language of our sense and memory lacks the vocabulary of such pain' (2010, Canto XXVIII).

Paradoxically, the presence of death was the cause of so much more death. It became a magnet, drawing the prisoner including doctors into the pit of despair, then into hopelessness and finally, in many cases, to suicide. Prisoners mostly became Muselmänner. The Jewish doctor working in Birkenau, Monowitz and the sub-labour camps never found respite from death. Death was hanging from the gallows at roll call. It was at selections. It was having one tablet for two patients so the doctor was the healer of one and became the executioner of the other. Death was on stretchers and in barrows when labour gangs returned after a day's work.

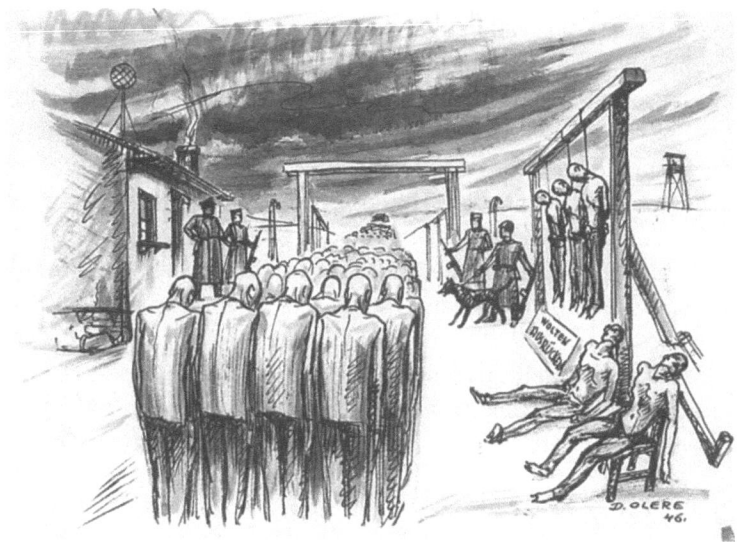

Fig. 21: Prisoners Going to Work. Olere and Oler (1998, 97).

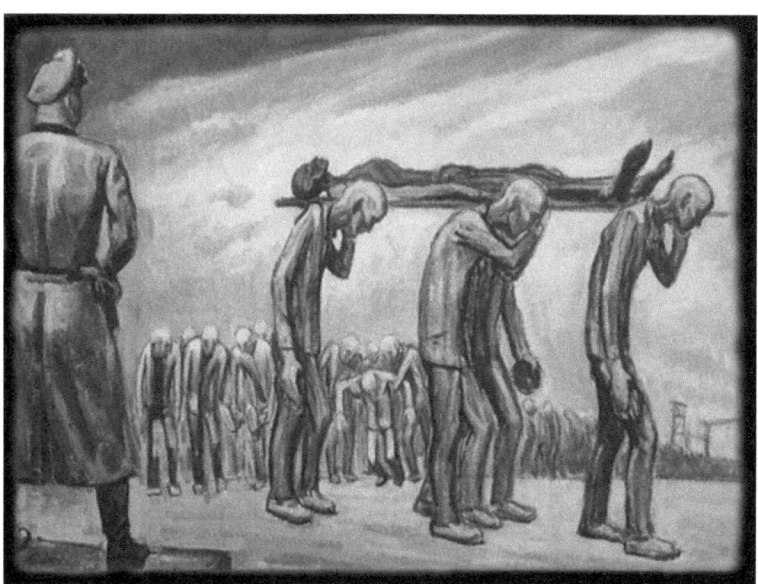

Fig. 22: Prisoners Returning to camp after a days' work. Olere and Oler (1998, 47).

When we left our place of work we always took with us several dozen dead comrades. Some had fallen under the clubs of the Kapos and the SS, while others had collapsed from exhaustion and starvation (Kraus & Kulka 1966, 29).

David Olere in Fig. 23 graphically lays bare the shocking unutterable and nefarious actions of the SS. Was the SS soldier on the left giving the Nazi salute in honor of Hitler and National Socialism or instructions to his fellow colleague. The actions led to the hysterical noises of mothers watching as their children, some still alive, were thrown into the fire pits. It was the smoke from the crematoria that worked 24 hours a day seven days a week burning bodies. The doctors were involved in or witnesses to selections, tended to the dying in epidemic blocks, and each morning removed the dead from the blocks. In addition, they treated Jewish prisoners injured at work and as a result of beatings by the SS and Kapos, and suffering from exhaustion and general illnesses. They faced dilemmas, ethical, personal and religious when attempting to treat and support the patients and to survive made choiceless choices and were subject to the human condition both of which forced them to make decisions and take actions that were both morally and professionally abhorrent.

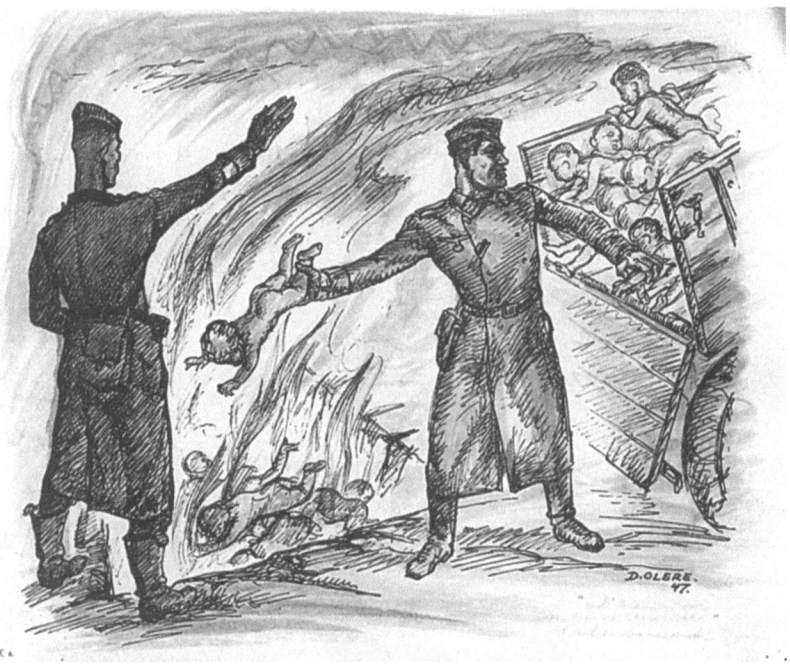

Fig. 23: SS throwing Children into Fire Pits. Olere and Oler (1998, 79).

Much is written about martyrs and heroes but 'mere' survivors appear to be of less interest. How did Senator John McCain survive six years as a prisoner of the Vietcong, during which he was held in a windowless cell without human contact apart from his guards? How did Terry Waite and Terry Andrews, both hostages of the Iranians, survive for six and five years respectively, in harsh primitive conditions? How did Gilad Shalit, a very young Israeli corporal held hostage by Hamas, survive for five years? They became famous household names during captivity their fate closely monitored by the respective governments, families and the media. Yet when they were released, they were treated more as celebrities than as individuals who had endured an intolerable and life-threatening existence. There appears to be no in-depth research on how they survived, on how they coped with no skin contact, little if any verbal communication or intellectual stimulation?

It would be meaningless and impossible to attempt to draw conclusions of how survival was possible by examining or interpreting the emotions of the survivor alone. Individual survivor's qualities cannot be compared, and the meaning of his or her words is not wholly comprehensible to the reader who has not had the experience of the victim. Take, for example, the connotations and symbolism of a single word: flame. The word flame to the survivor of Auschwitz may mean images of burning pits and hysterical screams or flickering flames reaching for the skies from the chimneys. To an ordinary person not subject to such conditions flame may conjure images of warmth from a log fire or cooking Sunday lunch over a gas fire. Jean Améry spoke of the ineffectiveness of words and the senselessness of attempting to describe the pain of when he was tortured

> Qualities of feeling are as incomparable as they are indescribable. They mark the limit of the capacity of language to communicate. If someone wanted to impart his physical pain, he would be forced to inflict it and thereby become a torturer himself. (Améry, 1986, 26)

In *Approaches to Auschwitz* (1987) Rubenstein and Roth refer to Auschwitz survivor Charlotte Delbo's trilogy of prose and poetry, *Auschwitz and After* (1995), in which they ask the question of what one is to do with the awareness that Auschwitz creates (Rubenstein & Roth 1987, 272). The scene that Delbo describes of her thirst quenching drink can be communicated to the reader but cannot be assimilated by him or her. When she plunged her face horse-like into a water bucket,

> Saliva returned to my mouth. The burning in my eyelids abated. Yours eyes burn when your tear ducts are dried up. My ears heard again. I was alive. (Delbo 1995, 72)

When, for example, she had chance to bathe in a stream, she noticed that, 'I took off my under-pants stiffened by the remnants of dried diarrhea ... and I was not sickened by the odor' (Delbo 1995, 72).

But what difference does telling this story make? Does the reader really understand or comprehend the feeling of exhilaration and relief or the pain that Delro expresses? Does the reader understand her emotional, psychological and physical condition? Levi, Wiesel and Améry agree that only survivors know and can understand the horror of the Holocaust. Des Pres writes clearly, 'an agony so massive should not be, indeed cannot be, reduced to a bit of datum in a theory.' However, survival of the camps and ghettoes, whether Auschwitz, Bergen-Belsen, Warsaw or others, should and must be researched, examined and written about even if we are only left with words and theories. Despite the truth in what Levi and Wiesel and other survivors say about the readers' impossibility to comprehend the emotions and feelings of the survivors and critics questioning the credibility and reliability of memoirs both must be chronicled for posterity.

My thesis is that survival of extreme adversity for an extended period depended on a number of factors unrelated to faith or miracles or any one specific element. It relied on a combination of extrinsic and intrinsic factors that enhanced the chances of surviving. A study of Holocaust survivors carried out by Peter Suedfeld that asked how they survived found that almost half of those questioned (49%) believed that luck, chance, fate or God contributed to survival (Suedfeld, 2003, 133).

> Many Holocaust narratives emphasize that unknowable forces (random chance, luck – or, for the religious, God's will) played a central part in whether one survived. Standing in one line rather than another, arriving early or late, volunteering or not, looking healthy or looking ill, speaking or not speaking German, could mean life or death, but never knew in advance which it would be. (Suedfeld, 2003, 133)

According to Dwork (1995, 93) survival must be attributed to nothing 'more – or less – than luck and fortuitous circumstances' While luck was a factor that may have saved a life at any one moment in time, it is inconceivable that it could be the universal explanation for survival over twelve months or in some cases two years or more. Some survivors answered it was because of a significant relationship, others because they were a cook or a scribe or they worked in Kanada. Age played a part. According to Suedfeld (2003, 133), the death rate for children was 90% while for adults it was 67%. Dwork argues that a strong will to live, involved 'failure or stupidity on the part of those who were murdered' (Dwork 1995, 93) yet fails to take into account or to justify the death of 90% of the children murdered by the Nazis. Then again there is the fantasy argument based on the 'just world' thesis that ones' outcomes is commensurate with their virtue and goodness. Interestingly, few of the survivors considered that their own personal qualities aided their survival. The work of Suedfeld, Fine and myself demonstrate through the application of different methods that reasons for how and why they survived are many and complex. Each reason given as to why was personal and how they survived could not be judged. There is a difference. My main focus as I have said is to present the hypothesis that survival of long term extreme adversity depends on the presence of a construct of survival of which there are three essential components that must work in unionism: Status, Personal traits and Defence mechanisms. The three components are driven by the will to survive.

8 Status

The difference between the normal and privileged prisoner exceeded even the most glaring differences in civil society. It was founded on the difference between status and its lack, a tolerable lifestyle and the struggle for basic survival.

Wolfgang Sofsky (1993, 125)

In today's so-called civilized society, we take many things for granted. We have enough to eat and drink. We have friends and relationships. We have freedom within laws and boundaries. We feel safe and secure as long as we are sensible. We have laws to protect us. We have a good enough health and medical system plus an adequate education system. We joke, laugh, go on holidays, we enjoy hobbies, sport, and we pray. We expect to see our children grow, find happiness and peace, and continue always to be good people. Our loved ones die and we can mourn. Most importantly we like to think we are treated as human beings. We don't feel privileged because that's our expectations.

Imagine another scenario: We are imprisoned in wooden huts, built as stables that could adequately house two hundred people, with approximately one thousand other prisoners. We are skeletal, shaven, tattooed ghosts of what we once were as human beings. We are woken at 5am every morning, usually next to a dead person, made to stand for hours in line to be counted in sub-zero temperatures in thin pyjama-type clothing. Some of us are without shoes, feet wrapped in paper. If we speak to anyone, we are beaten or shot. By the time a count has been completed, more of us have died and so, in an obsession with accuracy, the counting is repeated again and again. Breakfast takes place. It consists of a slice of mouldy bread and half a cup of putrid tea or coffee. We are so desperately hungry we attempt to steal the food from Muselmänner. We are allowed to go to the toilet once and for a limited period and then soil others and ourselves around us. We live in shame. We have no friends and have lost all trust in everything and everybody. We know we've been abandoned and are doomed. We feel sick but dare not go to the infirmary or hospital, because we know that these places are the anterooms to the gas chambers. So we go to work and know this will probably be the day we may return on a stretcher or in a wheelbarrow, dead from exhaustion, injury or beaten to death. Nobody will mourn us, or even care. We are no longer human; we are dispensable tools.

Starvation brings many to the point where we become preying animals. When life is at stake, everything is at stake. No matter how depraved, nothing is spared to get that last crumb of bread or drip of watery disgusting soup. It leads to fathers scratching, kicking and beating sons or brothers beating and even killing

https://doi.org/10.1515/9783110598216-013

brothers to get food. Herbert Bloch recounts the confession of a woman driven by self-preservation:

> I decided I wanted to live. Nothing else counted. I would have stolen from husband, child, parent, in order to accomplish this ... I ... devoted every fibre of my being to those things that would make that possible. Every day ... I had an objective: stealing a sweater, bargain for a blanket ... for an extra bowl of soup ... do something that I could survive ... I would remain close to those who were too far gone or too weak to eat their meagre ration of Ersatz-Kaffee or soup, and instead of pressing them to eat so that they might exist, I would eagerly take it from them and wolf it down, if they gave the slightest evidence that the effort for them was too great. (Bloch 1947)

Survivor Elie Wiesel was faced with a terrible dilemma when his father was seriously ill and he was likely to die. He and his father had a close relationship and were dependent on each other but a Blockältester tried to shake that relationship:

> The doctor cannot do anything more for him and neither should you. He placed his big, hairy hand on my shoulder and added, listen to me, kid. Don't forget you are in a concentration camp. In this place it is every man for him (sic) and you cannot think of others. Not even your father. In this place there is no such thing as a father, brother, friend. Each of us lives and dies alone. Let me give you good advice. Stop giving your ration of bread and soup to your old father. You cannot help him anymore ... in fact you should be getting his rations. I listened to him without interrupting. (Wiesel 2006, 128)

The advice given was arguably in his interests and Wiesel did consider keeping his father's rations for himself, but he felt guilty at having these thoughts and ran to get some soup for his father. He was not going to cross the line from human being to animal. His relationship and love for his father was paramount.

Freezing to death was as common as starvation, and again prisoners would use every means to survive, to get protective clothing. Properly fitting shoes were essential: If too small or large or, even worse, odd, they caused sores that would fester, crippling the prisoner eventually preventing him or her from working that would mean a death sentence. It is clear that conditions for the doctor and the ordinary prisoner were different. Prisoner Charlotte Delbro recalls the experience of rollcalls:

> Standing motionless since the middle of the night we had grown so heavy on our legs that we sank into the earth, the ice, unable to fight off the numbness. The cold bruised our temples, our jaws, making us feel that our bones were about to break our craniums to burst. We had given up hopping from one foot to the other, tapping our heels, rubbing our palms together. Exhausting exercises. We did not move. The will to struggle and endure, life itself, had taken refuge in a shrunken part of our bodies, somewhere in the immediate periphery of our hearts. We stood there motionless, several thousand women speaking a variety of

languages from all over, huddled together, heads bowed under the snow's stinging blasts. We stood motionless, reduced to our heartbeats.(Delbo 1995, 25)

Nyiszli provides a similarly sombre picture of roll call, but note how he refers to 'they' rather than 'we':

Night silence ended at three in the morning, just before dawn. Functionary prisoners woke their wretched fellow inmates with truncheons. They were all driven out of the barracks and made to stand in rank and file. Thus began one of the most inhuman items on the concentration camp's daily schedule, roll call ... All this lasted for hours on end. Frequently, prisoners could be counted and recounted in reverse order, moved from the front to the back and then vice versa as many as fifteen times. If one of the lines wasn't straight, all the inmates of the barracks were made to crouch with arms raised for half an hour. Their legs would wobble from exhaustion ... The thin cotton uniforms offered no protection against the rain or cold. Moreover, roll call always began at dawn and did not end before 7, when the SS-men arrived. (Nyiszli 1993, 17)

Nyiszli, who worked for the infamous Josef Mengele, did not live the life of an ordinary prisoner nor was it similar to the life of other Jewish doctors. There was nothing extraordinary in Nyiszli being assigned to a hospital but what were unusual were the conditions in which he worked and lived. He wore civilian clothes that gave him the outward appearance of a human being (Nyiszli 1993, 45). In his memoirs he speaks openly of the relatively luxurious conditions he enjoyed:

I drank some tea spiked with rum. After a few glasses I managed to relax. My mind cleared and freed itself of the unpleasant thoughts that had been plaguing it ... pleasant warmth penetrated me: the voluptuous effects of the alcohol, comforting as the caress of a mother's hand. The cigarettes we were smoking had also been imported from Hungary. In the camp proper a single cigarette was worth a ration of bread: here on the table lay hundreds of packages. (Nyiszli 1993, 45)

His description of his living conditions is disturbingly similar to that of SS Dr Johann Paul Kremer who describes his Sunday dinner in his diary, 'Today an excellent Sunday dinner: tomato soup, one half chicken with potatoes and red cabbage (20 grams of fat), dessert and magnificent vanilla ice cream' (Schlesak 2001).

But one of the darker sides to Nyiszli's position was his responsibility as doctor to crematoria SS personnel (about 120 men) and the Sonderkommando[67] (about 860 prisoners). He was in the bowels of hell, not only witness to the final fate of

---

67 *Sonderkommander* were prisoners selected to work in the crematorium placing the dead bodies from the gas chambers into the ovens and cleaning the human ashes from the ovens making way for the next batch of bodies. The prisoners selected were provided with the excellent food, proper clothing, accommodation and luxuries including an abundance of alcohol and cigarettes.

the Jewish prisoners, but coping with the human condition of the members of the Sonderkommando, who became instruments of the final desecration of the Jews in Auschwitz. Nyiszli's living conditions were exceptional but with good reason. As is now known, most Jewish doctors, such as Vaisman, Perl, Adelsberger, Brewda, Grunwald, and others did not enjoy such conditions but they did receive enough food and clothing and shelter to survive. They had the opportunity to get additional food and medicines on the black market, usually from Kanada. Some even had 'private' patients, mostly Kapos and Blocovas, who paid them in food and clothing for their services.[68] Obviously health was an important factor thus unsurprisingly the doctors represented a relatively large proportion of the inmates who survived, as Primo Levi submits:

> The privileged prisoners were a minority within the Lager population, but they represent a potent majority among survivors; in fact, even if one does not take into account the hard labor, the beatings, the cold, the illnesses, it must be remembered that the food ration was decisively insufficient even for the most frugal prisoner ... physiological reserves of the organism being consumed in two or three months, death by hunger, or by diseases induced by hunger, were the prisoner's normal destiny. This could be avoided only with additional food, and to obtain it a large or small privilege was necessary; in other words, a way, granted or conquered, astute or violent, licit or illicit, to lift oneself above the norm. (Levi 1989, 26)

Levi's comments is reinforced by Cohen and Micheels who note that doctors' privileges also exempted them from other hardships such as roll call. Cohen writes:

> In the camp we really lived a life apart. The life of doctors, who didn't have to go out and stand on the parade ground, who didn't go outdoors in all weathers, didn't have to stand outside in thin suits from half-past five in the morning till eight at night ...we got good food, of course. I say 'of course' – but it was a fact. You looked after yourself. The soup had to be stirred, but you can stir it vertically and you can stir it horizontally. The fat was on the top and the thick lumps underneath. (Cohen 1973, 97)

Micheels recalls:

> We had little to do with the other parts of the camp. We even had our own informal morning and evening roll calls: ten or fifteen people would gather between the blocks of the hospital nonchalantly. There was none of the rigid drill atmosphere of the rest of the camp, in which even the bodies of inmates who had died while working had to be carried to roll call. Our food was also superior. We got at least two bowls of soup and frequently a sort of farina as

---

Unfortunately after three months they were gassed and burned in the ovens and replaced by another batch of prisoners. This ritual was repeated every three months.

68 Private patients were both privileged and prominents who had access to food and clothing and paid for medical treatment, medicine and supplies in food and clothing.

well ... sometimes during the day we could sneak in a brief nap, an unbelievable luxury. (Micheels 1989, 70)

While the normal prisoner in Birkenau slept on a filthy straw mattress covered in excrement and vomit shared with up to five other prisoners, Nyiszli slept in a bed with sheets in the doctor's room of Block 12. He ate breakfast in a common room with fellow doctors and was spared the torturous and mind numbing roll calls.

Here reveille was at seven in the morning. The doctors, including myself, and the entire hospital staff assembled outside the barracks. The SS checked the number of those present, but it didn't take longer than two or three minutes ... We ate breakfast in the doctor's room, where I got to know my colleagues. (Nyiszli 1993, 18)

Micheels was shocked by the social demarcation between the prisoner doctor and ordinary prisoners.

When I began to know more people in and around the hospital, I realized that as a doctor-nurse I was sort of upper-middle-class in the camp society. As a member of the staff I received a double ration of soup and occasionally some extra bread. The better fed I looked, the more authority I seemed to have. It was important to husband one's energy. I managed, following the example of my veteran co-nurse, to sneak a little after-lunch nap in a corner...a strange feeling of immunity seemed to envelope me that was reinforced by my somewhat exceptional situation, my contact with Nora [his wife], my work indoors, signs that the camp conditions had improved. (Micheels 1989, 81)

Thus, the basic key to survival in Auschwitz is what I call the 'status,' of privilege, whereby a prisoner's position in the camp system that afforded him or her privileges essentially made the difference between life and death as a Jew in Auschwitz. Doctors also had the opportunity to form relationships with prisoners, patients, nurses, and other doctors and to work in groups, a form of socialization. They were also not as vulnerable to beatings and execution as the normal prisoners.

As doctors, they attempted to carry out their jobs as healers and carers. That gave them a meaning and purpose to life in the camp. Although their position inarguably increased their exposure to infectious disease – and many died as a result of contact with such patients – it is obvious that better conditions afforded them a better premise for health and protection against disease. In the case of Nyiszli, Micheels and Cohen, there appears to be no embarrassment or guilt expressed or seemingly felt in accepting these better conditions and luxuries. Nyiszli's memoirs give the impression that for him working with Mengele was business as usual. He could rationalize his work on the dissection of the bodies of young children murdered by the Nazi doctors and took pride in demonstrating his skills to prisoner and SS doctors. Although Micheels aims

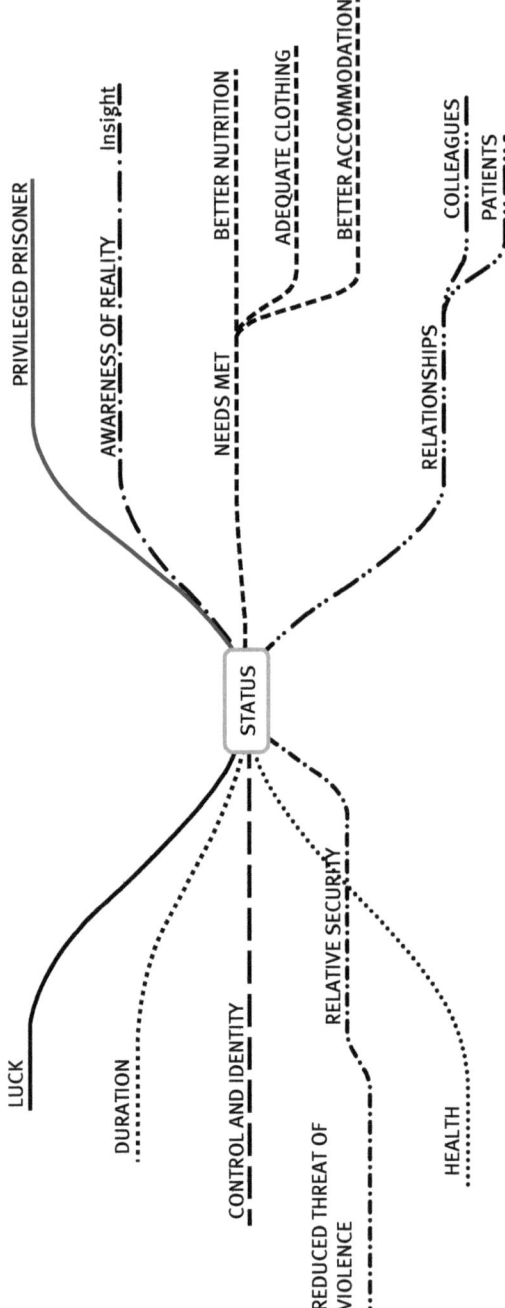

Fig. 24: Status.

were more modest he was cognisant of his position and the benefits it brought and he continually sought any place or work that allowed him some degree of safety and protection.

In order for the Jewish doctor to survive, a number of physical and emotional needs had to be met. We have already addressed the more physical fruits of 'status' but emotional wellbeing was essential. The sight of Muselmänner was a constant reminder of despair, depression and death. Jewish doctors were at the epicentre of the inhumanity that impregnated the camp; they witnessed the full spectrum of barbarism, more so than ordinary prisoners. From that perspective, the doctor was potentially the most vulnerable and required strong defences. The defences I am referring to are those that fulfil normal human needs and expectations such as relationships, security from physical and psychological harm, personal identity, individuality, control and effectiveness.

According to social scientist Jon Allen (2005, 115), 'relationships are the single most important source of satisfaction in life.' He argues that when people feel threatened or have experienced trauma, they feel 'a need to seek security in the safe haven of attachment' (Allen 2005, 115). The Nazis' strategy of isolating the ordinary prisoner – separating them from family and friends, and mixing nationalities in camps and blocks thereby making it almost impossible to communicate because of the language barriers – broke the ties of relationships. Levi maintains that communicating increased prisoners' slim chances of survival. According to Bettelheim most prisoners lived a very solitary life with few if any friends and could only be referred to as acquaintances:

> These were not real friends; they were companions at work, and more often in misery. But while misery loves company, it does not make for friendships. Genuine attachment cannot grow in a barren field of experience nourished only by emotions of frustration and despair. Jewish doctors had the opportunity to form relationships that were essential for their self-esteem and enabled them to regulate stress. (Bettelheim 1960)

Dr. Margita Schwalbova in her memoirs acknowledges that she was only able to function as a career in Auschwitz by working with other colleagues:

> Initially my colleagues in the Revier were German political prisoners, most of them communists, who had been imprisoned for many years ...from Czechoslovakia, there were the doctors or medical students: Ena Weiss, Edith Bock, Greta Reisfeld, Zlattner and the nurses ...later on, transports from all over occupied Europe arrived and additional personnel was admitted to the Revier. For example the women doctors, Zdenka Nedved, Margita Ernyei, Danielle Casanova, May Pollitzer, Adelaide Hautval ...all of them, without exception, gave all their energy, knowledge and courage to the battle to save human lives. (Shelley 1986, 16)

Louis Micheels describes his relationship with Dorus in the camp:

> He was about ten years older than I and quite mature, with a philosophical streak and a very special sense of humour that was almost as valuable as bread. My relationship with him and a select few ... became a kind of haven outside the Nazi grasp. (Micheels 1989, 86)

Micheels highlights the importance of this and other relationships in giving him a sense of being human:

> Where the human qualities and values could be preserved in a small enclave ... such a bond was essential as a protection against losing all traces of civilized behaviour and with them a true sense and reason for survival. (Micheels 1989, 81)

Lucie Adelsberger recalls the relationship that was established between her and two girl prisoners:

> The two girls shared the same bed; they got accustomed to each other and became like twins. They spoiled me rotten with all sorts of kindnesses, from polishing shoes to sewing on buttons. On one such occasion I let slip, 'You two care for me like a mother,' whereupon one of them declared herself my mother and the other my grandmother from that moment on. (Adelsberger 1969, 99)

In this regard, there was a common thread linking prisoners of the Holocaust to those in other circumstances of captivity such as prisoners of war. According to Lieutenant Colonel Bobby D Wagnon of the US armed forces, communication in a POW society serves three main roles:

> First it makes possible social interaction, second facilitates group dynamics and third serves as a necessary tool for socialization and indoctrination of new members ... conclusion already drawn is that strong communication ties among Vietnam war POW's [sic] were a primary factor in preventing the psychological breakdowns that were common ... where few such ties exist. (Wagnon 1976)

The experiences of POWs during the Vietnam and Korean wars and memoirs by hostages, held by Iranians in the 1970s and 80s, suggest contact with fellow prisoners, was critical. Senator John McCain, says the following:

> As far as this business of solitary confinement goes – the most important thing for survival is communication with someone, even if it's only a wave or a wink, a tap on the wall, or to have a guy put his thumb up. It makes all the difference. (McCain 2008)

Terry Anderson, felt extreme isolation. He suffered depression and missed the company of other people. 'Somehow, I can't seem to focus my mind. It's been a long time since I felt that touch, that closeness I long for' (Anderson 1993, 181). His excitement he felt on establishing contact with two new prisoners is palpable:

Hallelujah! We've established contact with two of the other prisoners...Tom spotted them looking out the little window of their cell across the way some days ago, waved and they waved back. (Anderson 1993, 181)

Terry Waite was isolated for some time, shackled to a wall and blindfolded when his captors entered his room or cell.

I am entombed, chained ... the damp walls rot around me, and my body, slowly ever so slowly, decays. Gently I place my hand on the wall and with my fingertips begin to tap. One-two-three. Silence. One-two-three. Once more, one-two-three. I wait. My breathing is labored, my body aches. One-two-three. One –two-three. A response! Can I be hearing things? There it is again: one-two-three. There is someone in the next room who is able to reach the dividing wall and respond to my signal. At long last someone to talk to. (Waite 1993, 326)

Lev Mishchenko was a prisoner for eight years and four months in Pechora, a notorious labour camp in the far north of Russia (Figes 2012). The elements, particularly the freezing winters, were life threatening and the living conditions primitive. The living space, as per Gulag regulations, was no more than 1.5 square meters per prisoner. The wooden houses had no running water or sanitary provision and the camp was without outside lighting, toilets or washing facilities. Water came from an open well. Lev entered Pechora in March 1946 and was released on July 17, 1954. His story of survival is one in which relationships played a crucial role. Prior to his imprisonment Lev met and fell in love with Svetlana, a fellow university student. Their love, demonstrated by the 1500 letters exchanged between the two during his incarceration, was life saving for him. According to Lev the letters gave him a reason to live. He also formed close relationships with fellow prisoners and free workers. Another key factor to his survival was his status as a valued worker in the wood-combine.

Relationships particularly with patients gave the doctors positive identity, which according to Staub (2003) is the need to have a well-developed sense of self and positive conception of who we are and who we want to be (self-esteem), which requires self-awareness and self-acceptance. The Jewish doctors assigned to hospitals, infirmaries and research areas were well respected by the patients. As doctors they had the opportunity to save patients, if only for brief respite from selections by fabricating medical records or hiding the prisoners. This gave the doctor a sense of worth and recognition of his or her positive contribution. The Greek Jewish girls subjected to gruesome experiments in Block 10 recalled and thus obviously appreciated the care and comfort Brewda gave them. Brewda also received respect as a doctor from SS doctors and prisoner functionaries. Nyiszli was respected by SS doctors for his skills as a pathologist and for his work in the dissection theatre. This activity has been criticised by some survivors such as Bettelheim but it gave him a sense of worth despite the odious and suggested co-operative nature of the work. Epstein, who was also recruited by Mengele, agreed to do experiments only if he could choose the subject. He chose to study noma, a gangrenous disease leading to tissue destruction of the face, especially the mouth and cheek, most common in gypsy children. That Mengele agreed to Epstein's conditions and that Epstein was successful in finding a cure for the disease were astounding achievements.[69] Recognition for their work gave the prisoner doctors self-esteem that in turn reinforced their sense of identity as human beings.

The ability to accept a new identity was crucial. After suffering many major losses; family, relationships, homes, a notable loss was the loss of identity; as a dentist, engineer, carpenter, businessman and so on. Most prisoners, successful in their chosen field whether a career or domestic duties became numbers and slave labourers. For most it became impossible to accept their new station in life. However, to survive despite everything that was happening to them they needed to quickly adapt to their new environment and accept their new identity.

The need to comprehend reality and being able to work within the boundaries of that reality is an important factor in understanding and accepting the environment one is over the short term. According Staub (2003, 57) we need 'to have an understanding of the people and the world (what they are like, how they operate) and of our place in the world.' The advantage Jewish doctors had compared to average prisoners is that they had more time to observe the world in which they lived. In being aware of the realities of the camp and the policies of the SS regarding the killing of every Jew in the camp, they could take every opportunity available to protect both themselves and their patients. Perl's experience with Mengele – after assuring her that pregnant women would be cared for if they disclosed their condition, they were in fact murdered – was a reality check. From that experience Perl realized Mengele could not be trusted and was dangerous. Brewda thought she was safe after being appointed chief doctor of Block 10 and given assurances she had complete authority, only to be sentenced to Block 11, the notorious punishment block for reasons unknown. She quickly became aware of the reality of SS promises.

Although as privileged prisoners, doctors faced many challenges and threats, they enjoyed a degree of security. What distinguished the Jewish doctor from his or her fellow prisoners was that the former was seldom subjected to the regular

---

69 Mengele subsequently presented a paper under his own name at a medical conference claiming to have found a cure for noma.

hospital selections, beatings, or physical and psychological torment.[70] This is not to say the Jewish doctors were not subject to punishment – the SS were a constant threat and the Polish and German prisoner doctors, who were generally antisemitic, used intimidation to protect of their positions. In his memoirs, Dr Berek Jakubowicz remembers the sense of relief and safety he felt on being appointed as a dentist in Auschwitz: 'I was given an elite camp suit, a sweater and a pair of real leather shoes ... I stopped being the dumb inmate and no longer needed to fear the Kapos or the foremen' (Jacobs 1959, 142). In a place where chaos ruled, the doctors and nurses tried to establish some degree of calm in the hospitals and infirmaries and to exert some control and effective management. This was difficult considering the injuries, illnesses and epidemics and the lack of equipment and medications. Realistically, the Jewish doctors did not have any degree of control, but when they achieved even the smallest of successes, it encouraged them to continue with their work.

Fabricating medical records or hiding patients would protect some from the gas chambers, as did organizing (stealing) medicine and clothing from Kanada. Unbeknownst to the SS, the doctors wrested some control over and were effective in their little corner of their world, which gave them a purpose in life and contributed to their self-esteem. Perl is a case in point; She saw her actions as being effective and felt she had some control over something that she saw as essential:

> In the end it was I who gave her a present – the present of her life – by destroying her passionately desired boy two days after his birth. Day after day I watched her condition develop, fearing the moment when it could be hidden no longer. I bandaged her abdomen, hid her with my body at roll call and hoped for a miracle which would save her and her baby...for two days and nights the spasms shook her poor, emaciated little body and I had to stand by, without drugs, without instruments to help her, listening to her moans, helpless. Around us, in the light of a few small candles I could see the thirteen hundred women of her barracks look down upon us from their cages, thirteen hundred death-masks with still enough life in them to feel pity ... then I could hide him no longer. I knew that if he was discovered, it would mean death to Yolanda (the mother) to myself and to all these pregnant women whom my skill could save. I took the warm little body in my hands, kissed the smooth face, caressed the long hair – and strangled him and buried his body under a mountain of corpses waiting to be cremated. (Perl 1984, 84)

---

70 The SS guards would often torture the prisoners for no specific reason. This included carting heavy rocks from one spot to another and back again for no reason except as a source of entertainment. This could continue for hours. Often during roll calls prisoners were required to kneel with hands above the head. They were required to stand in sub-zero temperatures for long periods. Those prisoners unable to comply were shot.

She did; Perl had control even over death. Micheels too had some control. Through his persistence, determination and his vast network of friends, he managed to contact Nora on an almost daily basis. When situations became toxic or threatening, he organized a transfer to another area or block. Epstein gained control by dictating to Mengele what experiments he was prepared to conduct and was eventually effective as he found a cure for the disease of noma. For a short period Brewda demanded respect from SS functionaries and received it, albeit reluctantly.

For a prisoner to escape the menace of emotional and mental sickness he or she needed to stay strong, just as Vaisman had told herself. To do that the prisoner needed to preserve his or her 'self', that is, his or her individuality. Michael Grodin (2010) says group behaviour tends to rely on diminishing the conscious individual personality, focusing thoughts and feelings in a common direction and giving emotion and the unconscious dominance over reason and judgment. Frankl argues that a person can lose everything except independence of thought. Retaining individuality and independence of thought was not common in Auschwitz but it was possible and, according to Frankl, central to maintaining a sense of humanity:

> A man's character became involved to the point that he was caught in a mental turmoil that threatened all the values he held and threw them into doubt. Under the influence of a world which no longer recognized the value of human life and dignity, which had robbed man of his will and made him an object to be exterminated...under this influence the personal ego finally suffered a loss of values. If the man in the concentration camp did not struggle against this in a last effort to save his self-respect, he lost the feeling of being an individual, a being with a mind, with inner freedom and personal value. He thought of himself then as only a part of an enormous mass of people; his existence descended to the level of animal life. (Frankl 1959, 70)

Some Jewish doctors managed to maintain their individuality. While this may not have made a significant difference directly, it gave them self-esteem and a sense of inner power allowing them to believe they had some independence. Another factor significant in the survival of Jewish doctors was the duration of imprisonment, which had both advantages and disadvantages, and the time of arrival. Jewish doctors who arrived in late 1942 through to 1944 had the time to adjust to the system and establish social contacts. They were assigned to the hospitals and infirmaries and had a greater opportunity to secure better positions rising to senior status. With time they became more familiar with the languages spoken and thus could understand orders and communicate with patients, non-Jewish doctors and the SS. They were better placed to form relationships with the Kapos and Blockälteste. On the other hand, the longer a Jewish doctor was working in the conditions and in contact with contagious diseases, the greater the chance of

Table 4: Jewish doctors: Age, Function in camp Period of Survival. (Czech 1990)

Name	DO Arrival	Age	Specialization	Incarceration period
Sperber	Apr-43	35	Gen Medicine	20
Vaisman	Jan-44	42	Gen Medicine	12
Perl	Mar-44	52	Gen Medicine	10
Nyiszli	May-44	43	Pathologist	8
Brewda	Aug-43	38	Gen Medicine	17
Fleck	May-43	47	Research	19
Epstein	May-43	46	Research	19
Cohen	Sep-43	34	Gen Medicine	16
Micheels	May-43	26	Research	19
Jakubowicz	Aug-43	43	Gen Medicine	16
Wolken	Jul-43	40	Gen Medicine	18
Fejkiel	Jul-43	43	Research	18
Bejlin	Jul-43	35	Gen Medicine	18
Seemanow	Feb-43	43	Research	22
Hautval	May-43	38	Gen Medicine	19
Grunwald	Apr-43	43	Gen Medicine	20
Adelsberger	May-43	48	Gen Medicine	19
Lejbus	Sep-42	36	Gen Medicine	28
Goldberg	May-42	32	Gen Medicine	31
Alex Grunwald	Sep-42	39	Gen Medicine	28
Kovatsh	Aug-42	47	Gen Medicine	29
Winter	Sep-42	46	Gen Medicine	28
Ladislau	Sep-42	37	Dentist	28
Freisinger	Oct-42	51	Gen Medicine	27
Rauchman	Mar-42	39	Gen Medicine	33
Franck	Sep-42	34	Gen Medicine	28
Lubicz	Sep-42	30	Gen Medicine	28
Imrene	Apr-42	45	Gen Medicine	8

dying. Jewish doctors who arrived in mid-1944 also had a better chance of survival because conditions in the camp had improved.

Survival was obviously dependent on individual state of health and wellbeing. In the cohort studied, the longest surviving Jewish doctor was Dr Rauchman, who arrived in March 1942. Generally, young healthy doctors possessed the physical qualities to withstand hardship better than older doctors. Doctors who arrived from transit centres or their hometown were healthier than those who arrived from ghettos and labour camps. However, while their prospects of surviving were marginally better, this did not necessarily translate to actual survival. Survival was also dependent on mental health. Arguably a young doctor may have been more susceptible to distress at the conditions and inhumanity than a more mature one. Certainly many Jewish doctors who were young and fit and 'enjoyed' better conditions were no more protected from disease than any other doctor or prisoner.

The final and most significant hurdle to surviving Auschwitz that prisoners faced was the death march. There can be no question that with the privileges of better protective clothing and marginally more food, the Jewish doctor had an advantage over other prisoners when commencing the march. However, the weather, physical exhaustion and the brutality of the SS eventually rendered all prisoners to the same condition – exhausted, frightened and in despair. Nonetheless there appears to be little distinction between men and women survivors.

Status is the first part of the construct. To survive a relatively long period in Auschwitz the prisoner had to have the status of a 'privileged' prisoner. Such status provided sufficient food and water to subsist, enough clothing for protection against the elements, and sanitary conditions and accommodation to assist them to fight and protect them from disease and illness. Their status provided other benefits such as the opportunity to form relationships and to experience positive feedback for their work, which increased their self-esteem. However, in conditions of extreme adversity, such as Auschwitz, having adequate food and clothing did not suffice. If the prisoner did not have the will to live or the personal traits to cope, he or she would perish.

9 Personal Traits

In extremity, the bare possibility of survival is not enough. There must also be a move beyond despair and self-pity to that fierce determination which survivors call up in themselves. To come through, to keep a living soul in a living body.

Terrence des Pres (1976)

Was status or privilege the pre-eminent factor for survival? According to my model the possession of certain personality traits was essential. While some personality traits would seem innate, the way we respond to situations both in thought/emotion/attitude and behaviour/action is determined by many factors, which are influenced by culture, education, religion, politics, childhood experiences, the nature/nurture relationship between child and parent, and the more complex family milieu. Thus, the doctors did not suddenly become positive, resilient, determined and hardy upon entering the most murderous camp in history. The doctors' behaviour was moulded by both nature and nurture that shaped their character and personality to provide them with coping skills to withstand and manage adversity.

In the case of the Jewish doctors studied here, there is a remarkable commonality to their early lives despite the stark differences in age, health, physical stamina, professional experience, language, community/culture, socioeconomic standing and mores. They were born thousands of miles apart in countries where the social and political history was characterized either by relative peace or by revolution and violence, yet they were similar: They were Jewish. Some, like Perl, came from observant families while others, such as Micheels, came from more liberal Jewish backgrounds. The most common aspect of their early lives was that they lived in Jewish communities where they could live in relative peace and safety. Their families were not wealthy, but they were successful. In their memoirs they described their childhoods and adolescence as a happy and exciting time enjoyed with family and friends. Their parents appear to have been disciplinarians who set clear boundaries, and expected and encouraged them to complete their education and follow higher education. They had contact with members of their extended family upon whom they could and often did rely. They felt loved, supported and secure, despite the discrimination and antisemitism that pervaded the villages and towns in which many of them lived. If they had not experienced antisemitism as a child, they certainly felt the full brunt of it once they attended medical school and went into medical practice. The love, support and security from family and community manifested positive attributes. These included self-esteem, resilience, determination and compassion. Their positive experiences during childhood and adolescence

https://doi.org/10.1515/9783110598216-014

shaped their personal traits and personalities that in turn formed their thinking patterns and behaviour.

As Professors Mayer and Faber from the University of New Hampshire maintain 'personality is the individual's master psychological system. It oversees and organizes mental subsystems, such as motives, thoughts and self-control' acting as a conductor that connects the mind and body (Mayer & Faber 2010, 94).

> Personality governs the connections between the mind on the one hand and the body and ongoing social situations on the other. For personality to function well, it must be in tune with all the environmental systems that surround it: the brain and the body that support personality, the stream of social situations that a person encounters and the groups to which that person belongs. (Mayer & Faber 2010, 94)

The early life of the Jewish doctors as portrayed in memoirs was one of relative calm, peace and security. Despite living under the dark clouds of discrimination and the foreboding presence of National Socialism, there appeared to be a belief that the status quo would remain and life would continue. The parents certainly were not consciously preparing themselves or their families for Armageddon. Their deportation to and arrival at Auschwitz, as well as all the events leading up to it, would have come as a shock, and the enormity of the crisis and resultant emotional and psychological impact probably left them physically and emotionally paralysed. Perl's response to the degradation and humiliation was not surprising. After suffering at the hands of Mengele and then yielding to the unbearable demands of a male prisoner, Perl fell into a pit of despair and feelings of guilt and self-loathing but, she recovered. She did not suddenly find the traits of resilience, hardiness, courage and determination to defy the SS; she had been developing these from the day she was born. Her success at school, her involvement in community and religious service, her achievement in convincing her father to give his blessing for her to study medicine, the triumph of being accepted into medical school and fulfilling her dream of becoming a doctor were all evidence of her determination, perseverance and resilience, in particular. Acceptance by her family and friends and the recognition of her successes gave her self-esteem, confidence and a positive attitude. In attempting to persuade her parents to escape the Nazis Perl demonstrated authority, responsibility and altruism. These are traits she possessed when she came to Auschwitz.

The profile of the Jewish doctor survivor is a mature person with an average age of 39 years, a well-educated professional primarily with experience in general medical practice, although some were specialists in their chosen field. Many, such as Vaisman, Perl and Micheels, came to Auschwitz from transit camps and the ghettoes and may have anticipated the atrocious conditions they would face. However, the reality of the camp was far beyond their expectations, and they knew they were in hell. Assigned to hospitals, the conditions and challenges they

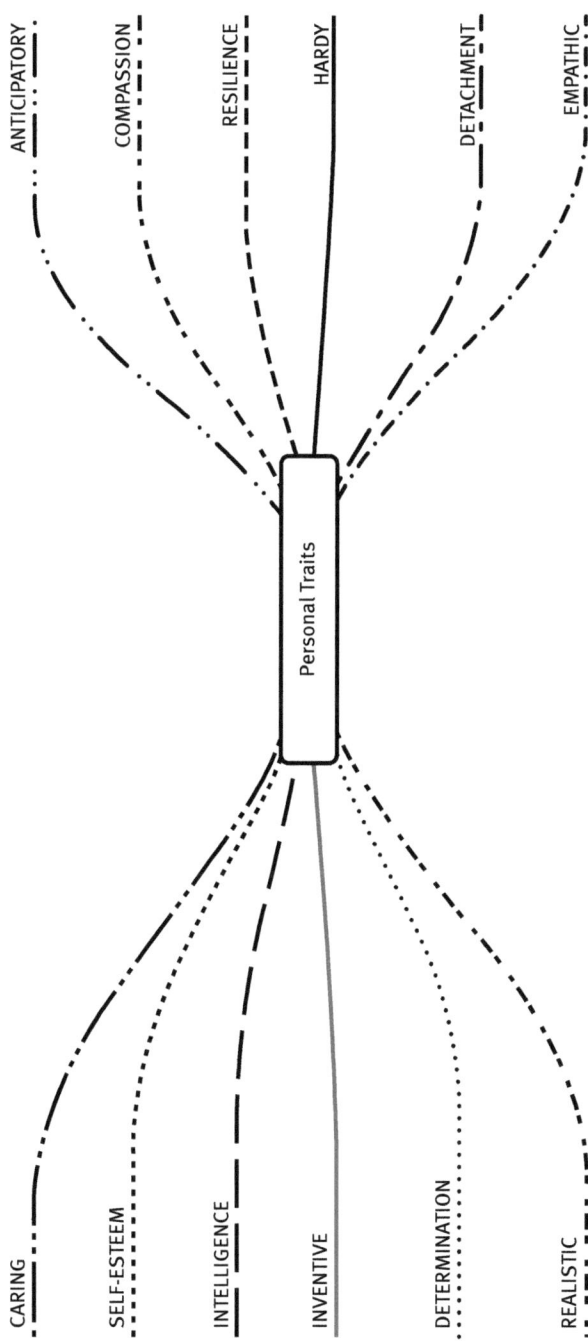

Fig. 25: Personal traits.

faced were not only beyond anything they had ever experienced they also presented religious, ethical and personal dilemmas.

We have already explored some of the emotional and psychological challenges that confronted the doctors: Grunwald continued to work knowing his family had perished before his eyes; Cohen was forced to murder fellow Jews; Brewda was witness to horrendous human experiments; and Perl was forced to drown babies, to name just a few. The reason for their actions and behaviours are both simple and complex. Primarily, as discussed in their individual profiles, they had a powerful will to live. However, there also existed a more complex set of reasons related to their personal traits and coping skills. Fig. 25 unveils the complexity of the personal traits that the survivors called upon. No single trait, such as resilience or inventiveness, was enough but a combination of a number some dominant others peripheral but important. Their ability to endure the conditions and cruelty in the camp and at the same time wrestle with the suffering and slow but inevitable capitulation of the prisoners is testimony to the powerful attributes possessed by the individual.

Jesse Prinz in his book *Beyond Human Nature: How Culture and Experience Shape Our Lives* (2011) presents the thesis that nurture is a major determinant of human behaviour. He contends that the influence of nature, or biology, as opposed to nurture has been 'oversold'. Prinz asserts that our behaviour, lifestyle, habits and values are strongly influenced by geography, history and I would add circumstances. Why are some people calm and controlled and others aggressive and irrational? Is it enough to just accept that it is a natural part of our makeup? Or are there other factors such as circumstances, experience or socialization? The behaviour of Jewish prisoners in Auschwitz to stay alive was anathema to that of their behaviour in their prior life. The prisoners' behaviour was determined by their circumstances, conditions, health, luck and other factors. Those who survived may have had additional factors such as personal traits and defence mechanisms (discussed in this section) that were both nature and nurture driven. Auschwitz is a case study of Prinz's position.

The most powerful personal trait in a time of adversity is resilience, the ability to bounce back after experiencing loss, failure, tragedy and trauma. According to Zautra, Hall and Murray (2010, 6), individual resilience 'may be defined by the amount of stress that a person can endure without a fundamental change in capacity that aims to give life meaning.' I have proffered a profound loss was that of identity which had to be accepted and replaced if the prisoner had any chance of surviving. The loss of self –esteem, strength of body and mind and self-control replaced by:

> Feelings of fear, vulnerability ... sadness over losses and weakness about not being able to control one's life or one's emotional reactions, contribute to feelings of defectiveness. (Marmar & Horowitz 1988, 96)

Kent and Davis address the issue of who is resilient by referring to the work of Rosenbaum and Covino, who identified ten characteristics of resilience exemplified by POWs in Vietnam:

> Optimism; altruism; having a moral compass or beliefs that cannot be shattered, faith and spirituality, a sense of humor, role models and a mission or meaning in life; facing fear; and training to become resilient. (Kent & Davis 2010, 428)

These observations have been replicated in other studies by Hoge, Austin and Pollack (2007) and Haglund, Nestadt, Cooper, Southwick and Charney (2007), who arrived at similar typologies. They identified a positive attitude of optimism, active rather than passive coping, cognitive flexibility, finding meaning, growth, social support, physical exercise and faith (Kent & Davis 2010, 428). Table 3 is a summary of the qualities, descriptions and findings of numerous studies of

Table 5: Resilience as qualities of human condition. Kent & Davis 2010, 429

Ten Qualities	Descriptions, findings	Authors
1. Positive emotions		Carver et al. (1993); Scheier et al. (1989); Folkman & Moskowitz (2000)
Opinion, hope, humor, see options, positive outcomes, humor, positive outcomes	Decrease stress related illness, increase well-being and health restorative, hope theory	Affleck & Tennen (1996)
2. Control		King et al. (1998); Soet et al. (2003); Kobasa (1979); Florian et al. (1995)
Locus of control, self-esteem and prime, control challenge and commitment, control over stressors	Lower levels of PTSD, components of hardiness	
3. Active coping, engagement, facing fear		Johnson et al. (2002); Beaton et al. (1999); Maddi (1999a); Rutter(1987);
Task-focused versus emotion-focused versus avoidant coping, avoidance versus engagement facing fear, leaving comfort zone, adaptive coping	Making plans versus venting denial, how you engage with risk exposure increases self-efficiency, courage, stress inoculation coping through emotional approach	Stanton et al. (2002); Meichenbaum (1985); Regehr et al. (2000)

(continued)

Table 5: (continued)

Ten Qualities	Descriptions, findings	Authors
Cognitive flexibility		Southwick et al. (2005); Manne et al. (2003); Wade et al. (2001); Seligman (2002)
Acceptance, problems temporary	Acceptance extreme hardship, tolerate highly stressfuln events	
Meaning and value inadversity		Tedeschi et al. (1998); Park et al. (1996)
Learning from crisis, posttraumatic growth	Value life, relationships	Tedeschi et al. (1998); Park et al. (1996)
Altruism		
Altruism, survivor mission, empathy, compassion	Successful adaptation, helping as coping, tragedy into activism	Bleuler (1984); Rachman (1979); Anderson & Anderson (2003);
Spirituality		
Making sense of tragedy, moral compass	Physical and emotionalprotective survival, health, core beliefs	McCullough et al. (2000);Koenig et al. (2004)
Training		
Previous experience of trauma	Training in stoicism, prior training in stressors; torture etc	Alvarez & Hunt (2005); Hagh-Shenas et al. (2005)

resilience. It shows that there are specific qualities that allow people to cope and survive traumatic events and gives descriptions and findings for each category of personal quality. Resilience, according to the table, embodies many fundamental traits that together enhance survival.

According to Fine (1991, 493), 'resilience is made operational by cognitive and behavioural coping skills and the recruitment of social support.' I have already emphasized that the Jewish doctors did not suddenly become resilient upon entering Auschwitz. Larzarus and Folkman (1984) suggest the skills did not come all at once but that resilience is acquired through a developmental process – a process of selecting from available alternatives and having persons reinforce the skills that are necessary to make coping possible. A long-term study by Werner (1990) revealed a key finding relevant to our Jewish doctors:

> There was a clear continuity, in that most participants who showed signs of resilience in adolescence remained resilient into adulthood, suggesting that core resources formed during childhood continue to promote resilience through various types of adversity into adulthood. (Werner 1990, 180)

The doctors' strengths and instinct to survive were germinated prior to Auschwitz but were cultivated by subsequent events. Before the war many had to struggle against antisemitism. The female doctors struggled against discrimination on the basis of sex in their desire to become doctors. At university they were discriminated against, ostracized and humiliated. The very fact they represented a disproportionate population of the medical community indicates their determination and resilience. Even within their own community, there was resistance to women becoming doctors, especially women from Orthodox and Ultra-Orthodox families. Perl's father was against her becoming a doctor on the grounds that her role and responsibilities were to be a mother and wife. According to Perl, her father was afraid she would abandon her religion if she pursued a career. Despite the pressure to forego her ambitions she persevered. Her sister also became a doctor.

Perl's drive to achieve her goals indicates she had commitment, faced challenges and had some control over stressors. King and Kobasa found that people with these qualities were hardy and had lower levels of PTSD (post-traumatic stress disorder). Perl, Wolkmen, Brewda and Epstein were all task-focused rather than emotion-focused. Johnson, Beaton, Maddi and Rutter found that people with these qualities were active rather than passive risk takers, able to handle stress, self-sufficient and had coping strategies. Micheels was determined not to give up in his attempts to escape the Nazis. He and his family were about to be dispossessed of all of their worldly goods, yet Micheels continued to seek a way out of the Nazis' clutches. Vaisman, after the death of her husband, fled to the south of France. She had suffered the loss of her husband and father and was separated from her family. Yet she endeavoured to escape the Nazis. She failed but in Auschwitz she vowed she would not surrender she would hold strong. She did, and not only up to the time of her liberation – she never forgave the German people:

> Dispositional attributes of the child, family cohesion and warmth and the use of external support systems by parents and children are mechanisms that buffer stress and promote resilient responses. Temperament, sex, intellectual ability, humour, empathy, social problem solving, social expressiveness and an inner locus of control have been found to influence adaptation under adverse conditions. (Garmezy 1985, 213)

As has already been discussed, the memoirs of Perl, Vaisman, Micheels, Brewda and Adelsberger tell similar stories of developing those sorts of buffers. The privilege of being a member of a loving and harmonious family is a start. It continued. What Prinz calls receiving a process of socialization – with emphasis on education, community service and morality – is fundamental to becoming a resilient adult. Resilience also is related to hardiness. The doctor was strong and healthy in constitution and was willing to undertake actions that involved risk and danger. Fine proposes that hardiness is characterized by challenge, commitment and control attributes (Fine, 1991). The Jewish doctors were challenged to accept or attempt to change toxic situations. Their actions gave the Jewish doctor a sense of control, which falls under the concept of mastery. According to Pauline Boss (2006), how and if one copes is influenced by a person's beliefs about the value of mastery, the ability to manage one's life, and his or her agency, the ability to exert power when needed to manage one's life. These particular survivors felt they had some control, that is, they could manage a part of their life, despite the dangers. At selection time in the hospitals, the Jewish doctors would hide patients or prepare them for inspection, for example redden the patient's cheeks. They would fabricate medical charts and results. And they would 'organize' (steal) medications and medical supplies. Leonard Pearlin (2005) calls mastery a liberating quality that frees people to be more experimental and forceful in dealing with life's threats.

Unlike in their previous life, the doctors could not rely upon their normal support systems such as family and friends when facing challenges. They depended solely their own coping skills and capacity. These do not, according to Fine, manifest as a constant state nor in a single act. Jewish doctors who survived an average of twenty months could not last by one single act of resilience. It was ongoing. Admittedly, the level of resourcefulness and determination might fluctuate, but to survive such conditions for a long period, strong traits had to be constantly in play. At times the survivors may have felt emotionally weak and vulnerable to a state of despair and helplessness, but after a short period their coping skills would have pulled them back into actively shaping their lives.

The resilience and hardiness of the doctors was balanced by empathy and what I would call self-sacrificing behaviour. I would also add the feelings of concern for as I discussed above there is a difference between the two each of which have pluses and minuses. Eisenberg refers to empathy as pro-social behaviour or voluntary behaviour that is intended to benefit another (Eisenberg, Valiente & Champion 2004, 388). According to Staub (2003) this is a personal characteristic whereby the individual has a positive view of human beings, caring about people's welfare and a feeling of personal responsibility for others. Staub examined a series of studies showing that people with a greater pro-social orientation helped more when someone was under physical and/or psychological stress. His own study found that the nature of the stress may signal the degree and type of help that is offered. Whether the help required demands initiative or suggest sacrifice depends on the circumstances. These may make it easy to avoid helping or exceedingly difficult in terms of embarrassment, social punishment and later shame or punishment (Staub 2003, 95).

Perl had a very strong sense of responsibility to save the lives of pregnant women by performing abortions. Her memoirs suggest she would have suffered terrible guilt and shame had she not come to the rescue of pregnant women.

Like most Jewish doctors, Brewda, Adelsberger and Vaisman worked tirelessly to comfort patients. Pro-social orientation may influence the way people look at or think about their responsibility to help. It is the feeling of responsibility for another's welfare that is the distinguishing feature, according to Staub depending:

> ... on how one thinks about such matters, one's interpretation of the meaning of a specific instance of another person's stress and one's judgment of the appropriate resolution of it (reaction to it) are likely to be affected. Depending on how one interprets such arousal-producing events as a person's distress, one's emotional reactions are less likely to be affected. (Staub 2003, 94)

By helping others, both self-esteem and positiveness are enhanced; 'After all, when they help, they act according to their ideals and therefore are maintaining a positive self-image' (Staub 2003, 95). Empathy linked to pro-social orientation is highly likely to evolve into either sympathy or personal distress (or both) with a sympathetic reaction often based on empathic sadness. But empathy can also lead to personal distress that is 'a self-focused, aversive affective reaction to the apprehension of another's emotion (e.g. discomfort, anxiety)' (Eisenberg, Valiente & Champion 2004, 388) The Jewish doctors were pro-socially oriented in that they cared and were willing to help, but under the circumstances they could not afford to be empathic. The conditions they faced were so distressing that to be effective as careers and healers over a relatively long period they needed to detach themselves from the suffering, pain and emotions of the patient rather than be empathic and emotionally involved. In a scene in the film about Perl's life *Out of the Ashes* (2004), Perl is shown, after the war, to be living in New York, when she is confronted by another survivor who was in the hospital in Auschwitz. The woman calls Perl a murderer because Perl refused to give her sister medication that she believes would have saved her sister's life. Perl obviously had sympathy but not empathy. She could not perform a miracle.

In order to be able to distinguish between sympathy and empathy and cope with the consequences, the doctor needed to have a sense of self, that is, to know who they were as a person. Many of the life and death decisions that had to be made were difficult and daunting, and the doctor needed to have the emotional and mental fortitude to know they were acting in the best interest of their patients. They had been subject to a process of humiliation and degradation that was meant to strip them of their identity including their self-worth and humanity. Despite these efforts on the part of the SS, the doctors stayed strong. Over time they gradually recovered their self-confidence, self-esteem, hardiness, ability to control negative behaviour and acceptance of their strengths and weaknesses. Their task was daunting if not impossible, but self-belief drove them to at least try. Perl knew her strengths and had self-belief that she could accomplish her goal of saving most pregnant women from the gas chambers. As a paediatrician Epstein believed that, given the opportunity by Mengele, he could successfully conduct scientific research that would help children. Nyiszli was confident he could work to Mengele's standards as a pathologist because he knew he was an expert in his field. Adelsberger was assigned to establish a hospital in the women's camp as was Brewda. Brewda was confident she could demand respect from the SS in Block 10. Persons with self-belief believe problems can be resolved by their own efforts rather than by 'fate' or 'luck.' It can be argued that people with self-belief know their strengths and are pro-active rather than re-active and this was the case with the Jewish doctors.

Self-belief only comes from self-understanding and the actions and behaviour of the doctors indicated that they were aware of their weakness and strengths. In other words, 'I believe in myself because I understand myself and I act knowing my weaknesses and strengths.' They had the personal resources to know who they were, to be able to define themselves. Micheels was aware of his weakness, his reliance on Nora. He was also constantly concerned about his relationship with the SS and afraid he would lose his status as a privileged prisoner. Because he knew he would not survive in a labour camp digging trenches, he was vigilant of any deterioration of his relationship with a Nazi doctor or the SS that might result in him losing his privileges. This is an example of avoidant coping. Adelsberger too knew her weaknesses. She knew she could not withstand beatings by the Kapos or SS if her roll count was incorrect, so she laboured to ensure that the counts were correct. The awareness of their weaknesses and strengths either protected the doctors or boosted their self-esteem, both of which facilitated survival.

Their self-esteem was also boosted by inventiveness and resourcefulness. To get things done they had to be confident, ingenious and cunning. They had to 'organize' medications and medical supplies, hide prisoners during selections, falsify medical records, release patients before and readmit them after the selections, carry out functions for the resistance movement in the camp and undertake many covert actions. Nyiszli recalls two women upon whom he was performing autopsies. The official records stated they died of heart failure but Mengele had reason to suspect otherwise. Nyiszli found they had typhoid but knowing such a finding would result in Mengele having all prisoners in the block from which the two women came murdered:

> I immediately decided that the findings Dr Mengele received would not confirm the diagnosis of typhoid. I would just not let it happen. Besides, the description of the symptoms was incomplete and the identification therefore open to question ... having proceeded with the dissection, I found that in both cases the small intestines had all the symptoms of the later stages of typhoid: they both had typical typhoid ulceration that was at least three weeks

old. Also in both cases the spleen was swollen. This was typhoid beyond doubt! ... My official diagnosis was colitis [inflammation] of the small intestine with extensive ulceration.
I gave Dr Mengele a virtual lecture of the difference between three-week-old typhoid ulceration and ulcers resulting from colitis. I also proved to him that the swelling of the spleen
was a frequent symptom of colitis of the intestines. (Nyiszli 1993, 72)

Mengele was furious with the doctors who had given an incorrect diagnosis and
threatened severe punishment. Nyiszli's report condemned those two prisoner
doctors but his actions saved hundreds of prisoners, at least in the short term.
I have questioned this action previously being careful not to pass judgement.
Providing Mengele with a false diagnosis may have temporarily saved the life of
hundreds of prisoners from being sent to the gas chambers because Mengele's
usual practice was to murder any prisoner who had contact with an infected
prisoner. However, the same prisoners may have been infected already and were
passing the virus to other prisoners. At the same time the prisoner doctors who
gave the correct diagnosis, typhus, were punished. Were they executed or sentenced to Block 11?

When the SS became aware that the prisoner doctors were deviating from or
sabotaging SS policy in an effort to save the lives of as many prisoners as possible during selections, the SS changed tactics. Each new policy forced the Jewish
doctor to invent new ways to deceive the SS. It became a battle of wits. The SS
doctors were determined to send a specific number of mostly Jewish prisoners to
their deaths while the Jewish doctor attempted to reduce that number to the least.
This attempt to save life was in reality just a game as all Jews had been sentenced
to death and the intention was that no Jew was going to leave the camp alive.

Another personal trait that is important and applies to the Jewish doctor is
intelligence. We have thus far concentrated on traits that can be related to socialization and the impact of family and early life, however, any discussion around
intelligence involves an aspect of nature versus nurture. It is not possible to
examine the influence of inherent factors because there is no evidence available.
It can only be assumed that as doctors they possessed a level of intelligence that
equipped them to cope with certain situations according to their inner strengths.
What has emerged since the latter part of the last century is the concept or state
of practical intelligence. This has been defined as the ability to adapt to life by
drawing upon life skills and common sense. In the case of the Jewish doctors,
skills, knowledge and experience may not have solved many of their problems.
This was particularly so since the most common problem, saving the life of a dying
patient, was not possible. Yet solving other problems, such as getting more medications and medical supplies or warmer bed covers, may require common sense,
life skills and much more. The doctors' memoirs suggest to me that: Micheels was

persuasive and manipulative; Perl was deceptive; Brewda was aggressive and a bully; and Samuel was manipulative and cunning. I do not say this to detract from them for these very characteristics both helped prisoners and saved the lives of the doctors themselves. On the other hand, the SS and members of the Einsatzgruppen[71] plied themselves with alcohol to deaden the nightmares and escape the emotional pain after taking part in Aktionen[72] in which hundreds of thousands of innocent Jews were murdered. However, alcohol did not do the job: The scenes were too distressing and affected the personal lives of those witnessing them. To solve the problem Himmler and the SS introduced industrialized gas chambers. The SS commenced using gas to kill the Jews because it shielded the members of the execution squads from stress and emotional pain. Apart from when an SS doctor selected which prisoners would die when, the process of killing was administered by the Jews themselves.

The Jewish doctor was at the epicentre of the pain and suffering with the job of selecting fellow Jews for execution or deciding who received medication or not. What did he or she have to stop the pain? Except for Nyiszli, as far as we know, the doctor most certainly did not have access to alcohol. They could not call upon family or friends for comfort or advice. To this point they were dependent on nature, inherent gifts, and nurture, life – long experiences, cultural norms and faith added with luck and with the blessings of status they almost had what was required to survive adversity over a relatively long period. The final piece in the puzzle was the use of defence mechanisms.

---

71 *Einsatzgruppen* Mobile units of the Security Police and SS Security Service that followed the German armies to Poland in 1939 and to the Soviet Union in June, 1941. Their charge was to kill all Jews as well as communist functionaries, the handicapped, institutionalized psychiatric patients, Gypsies and others considered undesirable by the Nazi state. They were supported by units of the uniformed German Order Police and often used auxiliaries (Ukrainian, Latvian, Lithuanian and Estonian volunteers). The victims were executed by mass shootings and buried in unmarked mass graves; later, the bodies were dug up and burned to cover evidence of what had occurred.
72 *Aktions* This word was a euphemism for the killing of Jews in the concentration camps after a *selection* took place or the rounding up of Jews in the towns and ghettos for transport to camps.

10 Defence Mechanisms

The mind's defences – like the body's immune mechanisms – protect us by providing a variety of illusions to filter pain and allow self-soothing.

George Vaillant (1992, 2)

During the five years of research for this book I kept returning to the same question: How did the doctors survive for such a long period? I had determined that status, health and reasonable conditions played a significant part. Likewise important were personal traits and coping skills. In a sense the extremities of the personal traits, coping skills and physical attributes needed to survive were extreme, if not abnormal. At the same time another factor that was in play and required an answer was a socio-psychological problem. These were the mental effects generated in the doctors after being exposed to continuous suffering and evilness. What tools did the doctors use to defend and protect themselves from such trauma? Bluhm maintains that 'the traumatic experience as well as the ensuring defense measures of the ego can be looked upon as typical phenomenon' (Bluhm 1999, 96). Did each doctor use a similar or a different mechanism to find respite?

Every doctor experienced trauma; however, the level that each could sustain depended on their own disposition. One could bear only slight changes in external conditions as traumatic yet another could withstand major changes without suffering major distraction. Micheels and Cohens' level of coping with trauma was less than that of Brewda or Perl. At the same time there was a difference between Micheels and Cohen. Micheels was most affected by the ceaselessness and unpredictability of the actions of the SS and Kapos while Brewda was in contempt of the same thugs. The memoirs reveal a number of doctors, such as Perl, Vaisman, Adelsberger and Micheels at some stage either attempted or considered suicide. Suicide and insanity were common in the first weeks of internment.

Vaillant (1992) observes that at times lives are intolerable to the point where reality is unbearable. Every adult and child experiences anxiety and fear in their life. To overcome these unpleasant feelings, we unconsciously use tools that distort reality in order to diminish anxiety and fears. The members of the SS and Einsatzgruppen[73] were given copious amounts of alcohol to cope with their participation in killing squads. These tools 'are often subsumed under the psychoanalytic term ego mechanisms of defence' (Vaillant 1992, 10). Vaillant argues that

---

73 Mobile forces of the Security Police and SS Security Service that followed the German armies through Eastern Europe killing all Jewish inhabitants

https://doi.org/10.1515/9783110598216-015

the use of unconscious defence mechanisms alter the perception of reality in a largely involuntary way. He argues that a defence is a descriptive metaphor for the temporary clouding of reality through thoughts, feelings and behaviours. Bluhm, proposes 'the mechanisms of defence … protects the individual from physical death and mental disintegration' (Bluhm 1999, 96). By the use of these defence mechanisms the person can escape or be distracted. They provide respite.

It is beneficial to distinguish between defence mechanisms and defence behaviour. Phebe Cramer distinguishes between the concept of defence mechanisms and defence behaviours. These are important notions when examining how the Jewish doctor coped. Cramer (2009, 4) defines defence mechanisms as 'constructs that denote a way of functioning of the mind', whereas defences are 'the specific behaviours, affects and ideas that serve defensive purposes'. She clarifies the difference between the defence mechanism and behaviour:

> Defence mechanisms, as theoretical abstractions used to describe the way the mind works, cannot be conscious. Defence mechanisms are theoretical constructs used to make assumptions about how the mind works … they are useful abstract formulations to explain behaviour that might otherwise be unintelligible. On the other hand, defence behaviours – that is, behaviours that serve defensive purposes – may be conscious or unconscious. (Cramer 2009, 4)

Under conditions of great stress, the use of defence mechanisms increases. As Cramer writes:

> [This] is a central tenet of defence mechanism theory. If the function of defences is to protect the person from excessive anxiety … then exposure to a situation that increases these reactions should result in an increase in defence use. (Cramer 2009, 6)

Based on this theory it could be argued that Perl, in aborting babies, used defence behaviour that was a conscious act. Her commitment to the abortions may have been a defence mechanism in the sense that this unconscious thinking protected her from intense anxiety and despair arising from the thought of the death of pregnant women and their babies and her inability to help. Her action in saving lives, however, was conscious behaviour arising out of her unconscious defence mechanism of sublimation, reacting to negative thoughts with positive actions. According to Bluhm:

> Indulgence in pleasant memories of the past, enjoyment of nature, discussions on all kinds of spiritual topics, and sometimes even extraordinary moral accomplishments – all these were immaterial satisfactions with which the inmates took refuge…their sense of beauty, their love of nature, was not destroyed in the camp. (Bluhm 1999, 96)

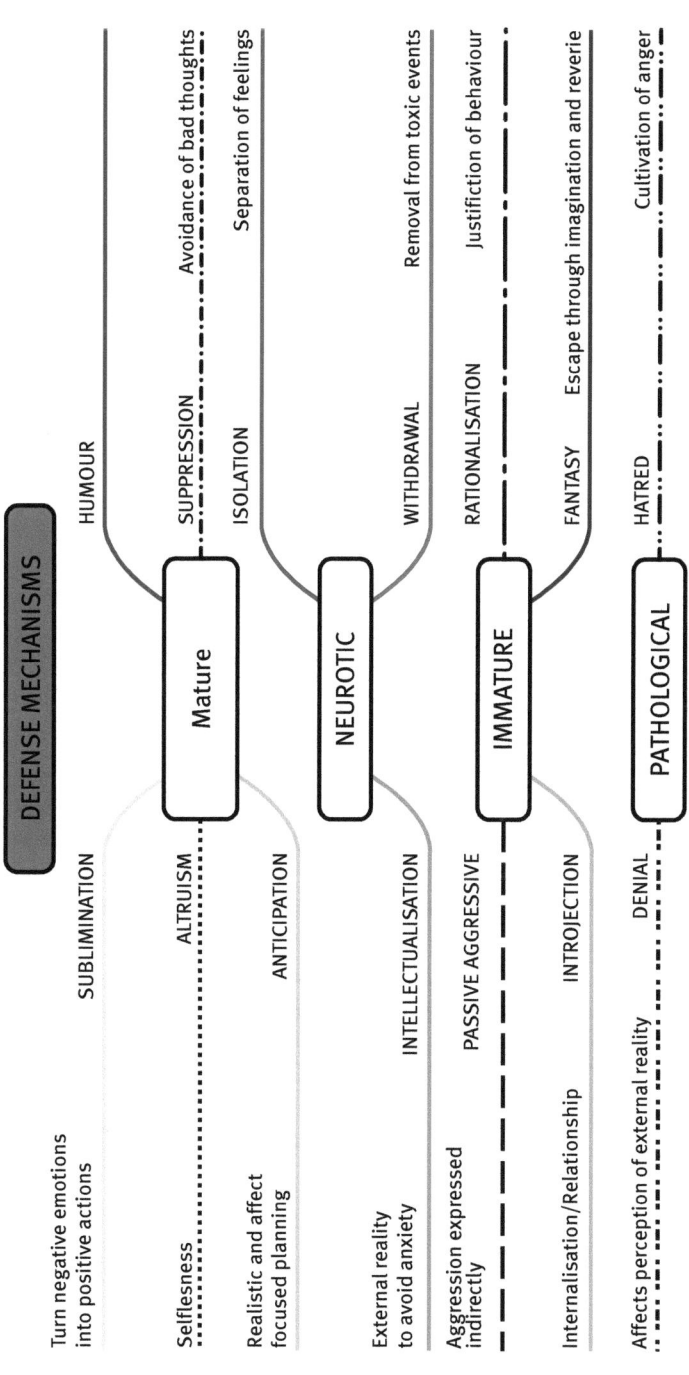

Defense mechanisms for survival. *R. W. Halpin.*

Fig. 26: Defence Mechanisms.

I have created a construct as shown in Fig. 26., based on categories presented by a number of psychiatrists and psychoanalysts such as Vaillant, Cramer, Anna and Sigmund Freud, Meissner, Kernberg and others. To create this model, I have used George Vaillant's categories of defence mechanisms – mature, neurotic, immature and pathological.

Defence mechanisms and behaviours allowed the Jewish doctor to use altruism, sublimation and anticipation to care for and protect the patients and to call upon unconscious mechanisms, such as rationalization, fantasy, hatred and passive aggression to care for and protect them. All of the defence mechanisms were part of the Jewish doctor's repertoire to some degree. Perl used defence mechanisms in all categories – altruism, sublimation, anticipation (mature), fantasy (immature), rationalization (neurotic) and hatred (pathological). The actions and commitment of Jewish doctors immersed them in a cause that reduced anxiety and increased self-esteem. In addition, it allowed them to continue to practice medicine, thus keeping their identity giving them some purpose in life whilst they continued to live. Their ability to concentrate on achieving a specific goal, purpose or cause to a certain extent deflected their attention from the culture of the camp, from the reality of the danger they faced and the insurmountable task they were attempting.

The distinguishing feature of life in an extermination camp compared to that in normal society is that prisoners in the former never had respite from anxiety and fear. In reality they never had the choice or opportunity to have relief. Additional food, better clothing, resilience and hardiness did not suffice. These did not offer protection against mental and psychological disintegration. Without a means to strengthen and at the same time protect ones emotional and psychological state of mind the doctors could not effectively treat and comfort patients, attempt to protect them during selections or experiments or make decisions and take actions that were in their own personal interest. Skodol defines these mechanisms as 'Automatic psychological processes that protect people against anxiety and awareness of internal or external stresses or dangers' (Skodol 2010, 115). Lichtenberg and Slap state:

> We take it as a given that the functioning of the defence mechanisms ... is triggered as a response to painful effects arising from drive-induced conflicts and from the vicissitudes of object relations. (Lichtenberg & Slap 1972, 781)

According to Vaillant:

> A clearly understood nomenclature of defences not only enables us to understand adaptation to stress; it also offers us a means of un-coding, of translating if you will, much of what seems irrational in human behaviour. (Vaillant 1992, 28)

In Freudian psychoanalytic theory, defence mechanisms are unconscious psychological strategies brought into play by various entities to cope with reality and to maintain self-image (Freud 1966). To paraphrase Sigmund Freud, the purpose of ego defence mechanisms is to protect the self from anxiety and stress or to provide a refuge from a situation in which one cannot otherwise cope. There is, however, an argument that Freud made errors in conceptualizing defences. Vaillant argues that Freud saw defences as only pathological and neurotic. Second, according to Vaillant, Freud believed that all pathogenic defences had their roots in childhood and saw defences as too exclusively related to sexual conflict. Finally, Vaillant believed Freud placed too much attention on a psychology of drives and too little on psychology of relationships (Vaillant 1992, 13). In this regard evidence confirms that sexual functioning almost ceased within a short time of entering the camp with Jewish women ceasing to menstruate and men losing sexual urges due traumatic shock (Bluhm 1999, 92). Relationships and the opportunity to be part of a group are positive influences on survival.

Once again, the memoirs tell us how defence mechanisms played a vital role in the survival of the doctors. Through the experiences and actions of the doctors, we can see that defences are not always pathological, as argued by Freud, but can be adaptive and a constructive human response. The examination of defence mechanisms in this study will concentrate on the work of Vaillant, the DSM-V (APA 2000), Sigmund and Anna Freud and other psychoanalysts. The examination will not be a comprehensive psychoanalytic study; it will be based on the behaviour of the doctors and the application of the theories of defence mechanisms to explain their behaviour.

In Vaillant's categorization, defences form a continuum based on their four psychoanalytical developmental levels.

Level I: pathological defences such as denial, distortion, splitting and delusional projection. Users of these mechanisms frequently appear irrational or mentally disturbed to others.

Level II: immature defences such as acting out, fantasy, idealization, passive aggression, projection, paranoia and somatization. While these mechanisms do occur in adults, they are more common in adolescents. People who use such defences are perceived as socially undesirable in that they are immature, difficult to deal with and out of touch with reality.

Level III: neurotic defences that include displacement, dissociation, hypochondriasis, isolation, rationalization, regression and repression. These defences have short-term advantages in coping but can often cause long-term problems when used as the primary style of coping

Level IV: mature defences are the healthiest and include altruism, anticipation, humour, Identification, suppression and sublimation.

In applying these categories to understand the behaviour of Jewish doctors, it is important to realize that there is a distinction between the behaviour of prisoners in a death camp and that of people in normal society. For example, Vaillant and others classify fantasy and passive aggression as immature defence mechanisms, denial as a pathological defence mechanism and rationalization as a neurotic defence mechanism. My argument is that in abnormal conditions under extreme adversity, these are normal or adaptive strategies. Jewish doctor Cohen and his patients would not have stayed alive had he not rationalized killing patients who were causing disturbances. Micheels and Nora may have fallen into a state of depression and eventual suicide had they not been able to dream and make plans for their future after Auschwitz. Cohen rationalized, a neurotic defence mechanism and Micheels was in denial, a pathological defence mechanism.

From individuals' memoirs I identified mature defence mechanisms as the most common in protecting the doctor against paralysing anxieties and fears. However, it is also obvious that the Jewish doctor used mechanisms within all categories to varying degrees. One of the most extraordinary gifts of the doctors was their altruism, their willingness to help others, and their commitment as doctors to do no harm. With altruism a person receives gratification either vicariously or from the response of others, those they are helping. Their memoirs disclose the willingness of Jewish doctors to care for and support their patients and the lengths to which they would go in terms of actions in order to protect and save them. Caring was an unconscious natural response while the actions were conscious and deliberate. In the camps the termination of pregnancies was something that occupied some of the female Jewish doctors. It gave their own lives meaning in as much as it gave them an opportunity to save another's life although at the cost of their child. Altruism gave the doctors the opportunity to do unto others as they would have done unto themselves. Vaillant argues that altruism leaves the self at least partly gratified; he goes on to say 'altruism resembles projection in that the self's feelings are attributed to the object; but with altruism, unlike projection, such attribution is empathically correct' (Vaillant 1992, 68).

The Jewish doctors invested in the lives of the sick and pregnant, instead of giving more attention to and protection of themselves (Freud 1966, 135). Performing abortions to save the life of the mother gave Perl personal satisfaction although painful to both her and the mother:

> After years and years of medical practice, childbirth was still to me the most beautiful, the greatest miracle of nature. I loved those newborn babies not as a doctor but as a mother and it was again and again my own child whom I killed to save the life of the woman. Every time when kneeling down in the mud, dirt and human excrement which covered the floor of the barracks to perform a delivery without instruments, without water, without the most

elementary requirements of hygiene, I prayed to God to help me save the mother ... And if I had not done it, both mother and child would have been cruelly murdered. (Perl 1948, 82)

Along with her devotion and commitment to pregnant prisoners and her intention to save the life of every mother, Perl's single mindedness and dedication to her cause subdued her distress and fears:

> I delivered women pregnant in the eighth, seventh, sixth, fifth month, always in a hurry, always with my five fingers, in the dark, under terrible conditions. Saving the life of the pregnant prisoner became an obsession ... but gradually the horror turned into revolt and this revolt shook me out of my lethargy and gave me a new incentive to live. (Perl 1982, 82)

She appears clear and detached but at the same time it is obvious she is angry. Adelsberger and Vaisman, who also performed abortions, identified with Perl. Findings by Bleuler, Rachman, Midlarsky, Anderson and Tedeschi found that in supporting patients, health care providers, in this instance Perl, Vaisman and Adelsberger, had fewer traumatic symptoms; thus the doctors used helping as a coping mechanism and employed their skills to turn tragedy into activism. The Jewish doctor valued life and was committed to caring and saving as many inmates as possible.

In conducting the autopsies on children (twins), Nyiszli believed he was protecting the corpses from incompetence and disrespect by SS and non-Jewish doctors. He would argue that there was a ritualism and medical procedure that respected the corpse and there was doubt that an SS doctor or non-Jewish doctor would follow this sacred edict. Epstein, who was literally forced, under threat of death, to undertake research, demanded and got certain conditions for the children who were involved in the research. Mengele allowed a special unit, the Nomaabteilung, to be set up in the hospital to conduct the work. Epstein felt he had triumphed over Mengele, for Epstein wanted to do ethical and scientific research that hopefully would contribute to medical science. Granting better conditions of nutrition in the form of fruit, vegetables, raw meat, medicine, sulfa formula[74] and vitamins succeeded in improving the health of the children. Epstein and his colleagues discovered important breakthroughs in treating Noma[75], [76] and witnessed significant improvement in sufferers of the disease.

---

74 Sulfa drugs were the first synthetic antibiotic to be put to clinical use
75 Noma is a " gangrenous affection of the mouth, especially attacking children in whom the constitution is alterered by bad hygiene and serious illness especially from eruptive fevers, beginning as an ulcer of the mucous membrane with with edema of the face extending from within out, rapidly destroying the soft tissues and the bone and almost quickly fatal (Auluck & Pai 2005).
76 In the camps noma was very common amongst gypsy children. Malnutrition, poor diet and diarrhoea are considered to be important risk factors for noma.

Frankl derived satisfaction from counselling prisoners who showed signs of giving up on life. This was not in Auschwitz but in Dachau. He presents as a person who was not afraid of death, however, he developed defence mechanisms that would distract him from the inhumanity and evil in which he was trapped. The memory and image of his wife, the welfare of his patients and fellow prisoners, and the belief that his mind was untouchable were Frankl's methods of resistance. He recalls the time he had the opportunity to escape:

> I made a quick last round of my patients, who were lying huddled on the rotten planks of wood on either side of the huts. I came to my only countryman, who was almost dying and whose life it had been my ambition to save in spite of his condition ... my comrade seemed to guess that something was wrong ... in a tired voice he asked me, You, too, are getting out? I denied it, but I found it difficult to avoid his sad look ... The unpleasant feeling that had gripped me as soon as I had told my friend I would escape with him became more intense. Suddenly I decided to take my fate into my own hands for once. I ran out of the hut and told my friend that I could not go with him. As soon as I had told him with finality that I had made up my mind to stay with my patients, the unhappy feeling left me ... I had gained an inward peace that I had never experienced before. I returned to the hut, sat down on the boards at my countryman's feet and tried to comfort him. Then I chatted with the others, trying to quiet them in their delirium. (Frankl 1959, 79)

What would seem to be a remarkable act of altruism gave him the very sense of gratification Vaillant proposed. In an effort for protection the doctors needed to anticipate and vigilantly watch for every move of the SS. Anticipation involves realistic and affect-focused planning for future discomfort (Vaillant, 1992, 71). Vaillant argues that in contrast to self-deception, anticipation spreads anxiety out over time. It involves the self-inoculation of taking one's affective pain in small anticipatory doses. According to Heinz Hartmann a pioneer of ego psychology,

> The familiar function of anticipating the future, orienting our actions according to it and correctly relating means and ends to each other ... it is an ego function and, surely, an adaptation process of the highest significance. (Hartman 1958, 43)

Successfully anticipating SS actions and reactions often saved lives. This is related to the personal quality of the Jewish doctor being aware of the reality of a situation. Perl learnt a tragic lesson in her initial contact with Mengele when he lied to her concerning the pregnant: She never trusted him or any Nazi after that experience. She became extremely vigilant and anticipatory. Micheels knew that his best chance for survival was to stay out of sight. But he also became vigilant of potential toxic or threatening situations and was pro-active in finding shelter and protection somewhere else. Nyiszli was wary of the unpredictable Mengele and well aware that his status of being a privileged prisoner was at risk if he misread the mood of the camp or Mengele. Anticipation of and preparation for selections gave the doctors a better opportunity to protect some patients. Frankl knew he could not endure heavy work for prolonged periods and curried favour with the SS guards and the Kapos to get favourable treatment. On the other hand, it could be said that Brewda did not anticipate the consequences of her outspokenness in protesting at unethical and unscientific operations. Nor did Samuel anticipate his execution when he apparently talked too much about Block 10 or when he decided not to complete surgery on women in sterilization experiments. Lack of anticipation could and did lead to death.

Another extraordinary quality of the Jewish doctor was the ability to rise above the culture of the camp and in a sense adopt a new life. Hans Loewald (1988) asserts that sublimation is passion transformed, that it 'denotes some sort of conversion or transmutation from a lower to a higher and presumably purer, state or plane of existence' (Loewald 1988, 12). Alfred Adler, the Austrian psychoanalyst and founder of Individual Psychology, called sublimation 'the healthy defence mechanism' because it produced beneficial outcomes for humanity. According to Vaillant (1992), sublimation provides impulse gratification by altering an objectionable aim or object into an acceptable one. It is the channelling of intra-psychic discomfort into constructive activity.

Sublimation was a powerful defence mechanism as it enabled the Jewish doctor to concentrate on a cause that required determination and courage and took time and energy. It became a passion. Using Loewald's definition: the Jewish doctor rose to a higher level of existence. He or she became committed to a cause.

> I had to remain alive. It was up to me to save all the pregnant women in Camp C from this infernal fate. It was up to me to save the life of the mothers, if there was no other way, then (sic) by destroying the life of their un-born children. (Perl 1984, 81)

In almost every case the Jewish doctor was committed to a cause that became an obsession, a neurotic defence mechanism. Out of outrage at the cruelty and inhumanity, the Hungarian Jewish doctor Otto Wolken became committed to recording data as proof of the atrocities. The act became an obsession and in so doing became a defence mechanism for his commitment gave him respite from the constant fear of the surrounding inhumanity and gave him purpose and the will to live. He methodically recorded the health statistics of the prisoner patients' weight, height, calorie intake and length of time in hospital. He kept comprehensive records of train arrivals and received information about the fate of the prisoners (see Appendices I). In one report he examines the fate of prisoners who arrived on fourteen cattle trains in mid-1942. The report concludes that there were 'systematic actions against certain groups of Jews' presumably on the basis of nationality, but that after five months in the camp, no more than five per cent of any transport was still alive. In Appendices I, page 225, there is a telegram from Heinrich Schwarz, labour chief in KL Auschwitz, concerning the fate of Jews arriving at the camp. An example of his work is Table 6 in which Wolken's report contains the same information in a similar format to that in Schwarz's telegram. It reveals by 1942, 8973 of the 9863 prisoners admitted from these 15 transports had been killed. The number of daily deaths depended largely on circumstances as was the case on June 16 during the visit of Himmler when no prisoner from the transports died yet on June 28, 189 prisoners died. The figures show that prisoners from Poland seem to have fared significantly better than those from Slovakia who were killed more quickly. This indicates that Wolken had access to these official communiqués. He was persistent and cunning and it is highly likely he fostered relationships to keep his obsession alive. I addressed the importance of relationships when looking at the benefit of becoming a privileged prisoner.

Table 6: The fate of Jewish prisoners as recorded by Dr Otto Wolken who arrived at Auschwitz over a three month period 1942.

Date of Arrival Auschwitz	Departure From	No. of Prisoners on Each Train	Prisoners Alive 15 Aug. 1942	% of Prisoners died by 15 August 1942
Apr-15	Slovakia	972	86	91%
19	Slovakia	464	10	98%
22	Slovakia	542	41	93%
Apr-29	Slovakia	442	23	
Apr-27	Slovakia	442	23	95%
Apr-29	Slovakia	423	20	95%
May-22	Slovakian prisoners transferred from Lublin	1000	52	94%
Jun-07	Paris	1000	217	78%
Jun-20	Slovakia	404	45	89%
Jun-24	Paris	933	186	80%
Jun-27	Poland	1000	557	44%
Jun-30	Poland	1004	702	30%
Jun-30	Slovakian prisoners transferred from Lublin	400	208	48%
Jul-04	Slovakia	264	69	70%
Jul-11	Slovakia	182	64	65%
Jul-17	Netherlands	651	428	30%

The internalization of the characteristics of a person or object with the hope of establishing or continuing a relationship is a defence mechanism in itself and referred to as introjection. Micheels used introjection when he lost contact with Nora. His feelings were directed to the mental image of Nora. In his memoirs he expressed his dependence on Nora, constantly thinking of her even when they were apart for a day. Although Micheels used other mechanisms such as fantasy and sublimation, where he transformed negative emotions into positive emotions through his love and dependency on Nora as well as anticipation, introjection was his mainstay. Samuel used introjection similarly in respect to his daughter. Her life was paramount and it was the image of her that he clung to and which drove him to continue to work for the SS.

A powerful defence mechanism that Vaisman used was hatred; she carried it with her until she died in Paris. Obviously, the Jewish doctors felt intense hatred of the SS. In Auschwitz hatred defended the prisoner against a depressing, humiliating situation. Kernberg has described hatred as a process called 'fixation to the trauma' (Kernberg 1991, 99). According to Kernberg hatred is not always pathological, that is, affected by emotional disorder. (Vitz & Mago, 1997, 64), writing on Kleinian psychodynamics of hatred, argues that when it is a response to an objective, real danger, a threat to the survival of self-and/or those one loves, hatred is a normal collaboration of rage aimed at eliminating that danger. This type of reaction is primarily considered justified anger. In these cases, hatred at its core is not affect but volition. Vitz maintains that hatred is a choice that under normal circumstances is never healthy, and that the person should work on a process of forgiveness. Jewish prisoners, however, endured extreme conditions in which anger and hatred were the norm. Forgiveness was not part of the prisoners' vocabulary. Vitz suggests that moral pride in one's self is defended by hatred. As did every prisoner in Auschwitz, Vaisman witnessed women, children and elderly people going to the gas chambers upon arrival and asked the following: 'How can we continue to live like this? It is only hatred that gives us strength and hope to see the Nazi regime collapse before our eyes' (Vaisman 2005, 58).

The following is a summary of the suggested defence mechanisms of individual doctors, including a description of those defence mechanism, along with sources of information.

The study of personal traits and defence mechanisms does have limitations when attempting to make theoretical distinctions. As stated previously, personal traits such as resilience, hardiness, determination, courage, defiance and self-esteem do not suddenly appear, they are developed one step at a time over a long period from early in life. Defence mechanisms are a reaction to toxic situations in which in the case of the Jewish doctors their very existence was at stake. It can be argued that some personal traits reinforce defence mechanisms. There are also crossovers between personal traits and defence mechanisms, such as with altruism and empathy, which can be categorized as both a personal trait and as a defence mechanism. Hatred could be considered a personal trait learnt from an early life of discrimination and abuse for Jewish, or a defence mechanism that came about because of the cruelty both experienced and witnessed. What is clear

Table 7: A Summary of defence mechanisms used by Jewish doctors as Survival tools.

Defence Mechanisms	Descriptions, findings	Sources
Anticipation – Mature Micheels, Vaisman, Adelsberger, Brewda	Anticipation or planning for future inner discomfort, insight, worry, anxiety	Vaillant 1992 Stanescu/ et al. 2005
Altruism – Mature Perl, Vaisman, Adelsberger, Brewda, Perl, Micheels,	Gratifying service to others to undergo a vicarious experience, helpful, considerate, caring	Vaillant, 1992 DSM-IV 2000
Altruism – Mature Perl, Vaisman, Adelsberger, Brewda, Perl, Micheels,	Gratifying service to others to undergo a vicarious experience, helpful, considerate, caring	Vaillant, 1992 DSM-IV 2000
Humour – Mature	Comedy to overtly express feelings without discomfort to others	Vaillant 1977, 1992
Suppression – Mature Jewish doctors	Avoiding thinking about disturbing experiences	Meissner 1970, Vaillant 1992
Denial – Psychotic Jewish doctors	Abolishing external reality, refusal to acknowledge pain of inner or outer reality	Vaillant, 1992
Hatred – Pathological Vaisman, Perl, Adelsberger	Self-righteous cultivation of anger, aggression, revenge, destruction, object relations (splitting)	Kernberg 1991
Rationalization – Immature Cohen, Perl	Rational explanations to justify behaviour and beliefs	DSM-IV 2000 Vaillant 1992
Passive-aggression – Immature All doctors	Direct or indirect aggression towards others	Vaillant 1992
Introjection –Immature Micheels	Internalization of characteristics of a loved object	Meissner 1970

is that to survive in the toxic culture of Auschwitz, prisoner doctors required resilience, determination and other personal traits to allow them to put into place the mechanisms that would provide both psychological and hopefully physical respite.

The answer to my question of why Jewish doctors went to so much trouble and risked their own lives to save a prisoner's life in an extermination camp is that it was one of their defence mechanisms. By committing their time, energy and life to treating, caring and comforting the patient they gave their lives meaning. They had dual responsibilities. As a doctor they had a commitment to the patient and as a person they had an innate commitment to themselves. They were performing a gratifying if admittedly hopeless service and at the same time in the majority of cases fought a losing battle to stay alive. The patient desperately needed the doctor but the doctor needed something far more illusive; respite from the suffering; emotional and psychological resilience and hardiness and other defences to cope.

Part V: **Anatomy of Survival**

One is never in another's place. Each individual is so complex an object that there is no point in trying to foresee his behaviour, all the more so in extreme situations; and neither is it possible to foresee one's own behaviour.

Primo Levi (1989, 43)

At the root of survival was the will to live. This was essential. It is my belief that survival was not haphazard or due to luck or happenstance but it was structured and integrated; that it was based on three pillars: status, personality traits and defence mechanisms.

The first component, status, consisted of having adequate food and clothing; the second, personal traits, consisted of possessing qualities such as resilience and hardiness; and the third component, consisted of using defence mechanisms such as, altruism, sublimation and hatred. Status was externally driven while personal traits and defence mechanisms were internal forces. Survival could only take place if all three components co-existed. If one component was missing survival was nigh impossible.

The Jewish doctors were aware that their status as a doctor, assigned to work in the hospitals and infirmaries, was fundamental to their survival. Lifton quotes unnamed prisoner doctors saying, 'if I were not in the hospital, [as a doctor] I'd be dead too'; 'for me to be a doctor has been lifesaving'; and, 'We survived because of our profession' (Lifton 2000, 218). The main instruments of death were lack of food and clothing. Deprivation of nourishment and inadequate clothing was part of a systematic program initiated by the SS to destroy the Jews mentally and physically, to bring them to their knees once they had lost all hope. Food was the essence of life. If prisoners could not get sufficient food, they starved to death. Lifton quotes a prisoner doctor saying, 'all those who survived Auschwitz lived from the food that was taken away from the others' (Lifton 2000, 218). History has shown that hundreds of thousands if not millions of people have starved to death. In the siege of Leningrad during World War II approximately 750,000 people died of starvation. Under Stalin and Mao's reigns of terror millions of people died of starvation. Irrespective of their standing in the community, of personal traits or commitment to a cause, without food, people die. Once resilient, determined and optimistic people become broken in spirit, emaciated in body and deranged in mind. Finally they give up on life. This is what happened to so many prisoners of Auschwitz.

As we have learnt survival was not dependent on food alone. The Jewish doctors had to confront personal, emotional and psychological torment and challenges. Being in a labour camp, the Jews were used as slaves and worked to a state of exhaustion that brought a painful and cruel death. The Jewish doctors were assigned to mend any sick and injured prisoners to get them back to work at which they finally met their death. The doctors in effect became a cog in the

https://doi.org/10.1515/9783110598216-016

wheel of death. How does a 'normal' person withstand the ceaseless conflict between life and death? Between everything a doctor believes and practices, to save a life, to what has become in reality, a participant in the killing process. It is at this point that their personal traits such as resilience and hardiness and other traits were needed to survive the horrific paradox of which they were part. Finally, to survive the doctors also needed some respite from the relentless inhumanity and depravation. They needed a brief period when they could indulge themselves in some activity that gave them meaning and a will to live. They needed defence mechanisms.

How did each doctor survive? Did they all depend equally on each pillar? Or did each depend differently according to their strengths and weaknesses? Once again the memoirs yielded the answer. Not every Jewish doctor had the same experiences. Most were assigned to Auschwitz-Birkenau, the largest camp that supplied labour and where the crematoriums and gas chambers were situated. Birkenau was the worst of the three camps where many of the doctors lived and worked. Their privileges amounted to receiving just enough food to survive and adequate clothing and shoes to withstand the elements. Other more fortunate Jewish doctors were assigned to research centres or blocks where human experiments were conducted. At these places the food, clothing and sleeping and working conditions were better than those in Birkenau or the satellite labour camps. Each Jewish doctor exhibited differing degrees of dependency on the three components for survival.

Louis Micheels

To survive, Micheels depended on the benefits of his status to a greater extent than on defence mechanisms or personality traits. His strong dependence on Nora was an immature defence mechanism (introjection). His main personality traits were resilience, determination and anticipation.

Micheels was largely dependent on the benefits of being a privileged prisoner. He worked in the Institute of Hygiene at Raisko for twelve months where on a comparative basis conditions were excellent. He commented that:

> In contrast to Birkenau, the camp and barracks were relatively clean, free of mud, with regular toilets, running water and no stench. Nourishment was inadequate, but there were enough extra supplies to sustain me. (Micheels 1989, 193)

Micheels used fantasy and denial as defence mechanisms when he and Nora would discuss their future after Auschwitz – making plans to marry, to follow

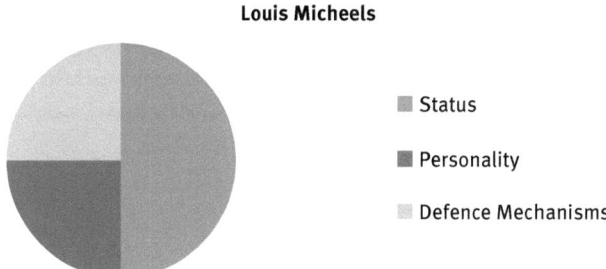

Fig. 27: Survival primarily dependent upon status.

their individual careers and have children. It could be argued his behaviour was immature, given that these fantasies took place in a sea of brutality and death. He believed Nora was his saviour and he was terrified that he would lose contact with her. He used introjection in which Nora was a loved object that involved the internalization of characteristics with the goal of establishing a close relationship.

Gisella Perl

The main components of survival for Perl were her mature defence mechanisms of altruism and sublimation based on her dedication and commitment to saving the lives of pregnant women. Significant factors for her survival also included strong personal traits of resilience, determination, hardiness and self-esteem. Status was a comparatively minor factor.

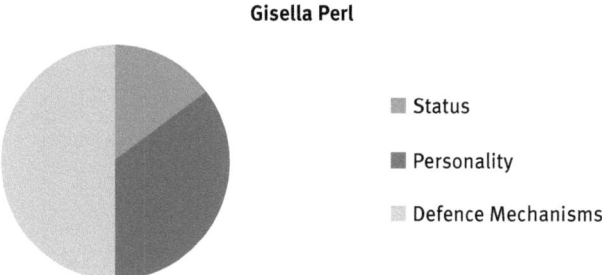

Fig. 28: Survival primarily dependent upon Defence Mechanisms and Personal Traits

She was selfless and committed to saving lives: altruism. She was vigilant and anticipatory: anticipation. She used sublimation in acknowledging her feelings and directing them toward a significant goal, saving pregnant women, so that satisfaction resulted both for her and her patient. Perl was passive aggressive when she acted against the SS by aborting babies despite the fact that this was strictly forbidden and could lead to her death. Her behaviour here could be considered a personality trait.

Sima Vaisman

Vaisman's major contributors to survival were her personal traits, of which the most prominent were resilience and hardiness. The defence mechanism of altruism played an important role, but hatred was the one that kept her focused and occupied. Status was of comparatively minor importance. Vaisman worked in Birkenau and endured the wretched conditions. She received better clothing and bedding and marginally more food than the prisoners in her block. But like Perl her conditions were woeful. Vaisman slept and had meals with the patients in her block and in doing so was in constant contact with patients suffering from deadly disease and illness. She was a resilient, hardy, mature and experienced doctor who could manage most situations and emergencies. She claimed she was determined to live to bear witness to the atrocities. Before the Holocaust she had lived through painful losses and had suffered antisemitism. These experiences helped to prepare her for the hardships of being a doctor in the camp.

In regard to defence mechanisms Vaisman's main tools were hatred and altruism. She had an intense hatred for the Nazis that it seems she carried with her after the war. She was altruistic in her selfless actions in caring and saving, or attempting to save, lives. Like Perl, she performed abortions to save the life of mothers. Vaisman presents herself as a woman of strength and honour and this is reflected in her life after Auschwitz.

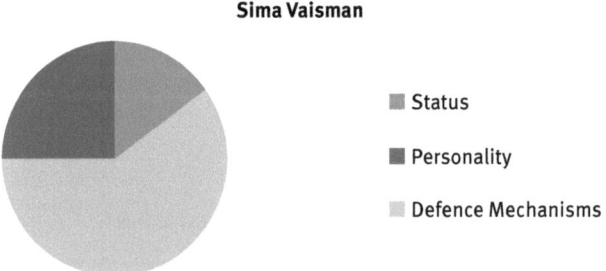

Sima Vaisman

- Status
- Personality
- Defence Mechanisms

Fig. 29: Survival primarily dependent upon Defence Mechanisms.

Alina Brewda

Brewda's survival was enhanced by strong personal traits of resilience, assertiveness, high self-esteem, pro-social skills, empathy and independence. Defence mechanisms such as sublimation and anticipation played a crucial role, as did her altruism in committing to protect and comfort Jewish women undergoing horrendous unethical, unscientific and murderous surgery. Status also contributed to her survival. She enjoyed better conditions working in Block 10, including adequate food and clothing, and there are witness reports of her enjoying certain luxuries. She demanded respect from her colleagues and refused to operate; this was accepted by the SS for a time.

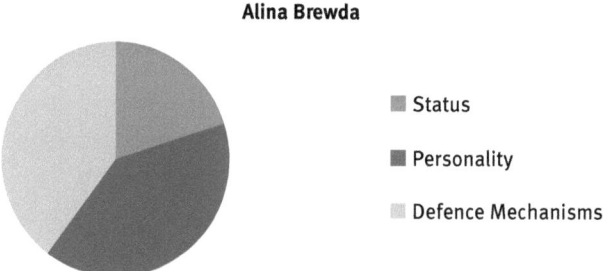

Fig. 30: Survival primarily dependent on Defence Mechanisms and Personal Traits.

Lucie Adelsberger

Adelsberger relied primarily upon her personality traits of resilience, hardiness, empathy and determination. Status did not play a major role, but she formed strong relationships with colleagues and patients. Like Perl, she used sublimation and altruism as defence mechanisms. She was committed to saving the lives of pregnant women and to the care of gypsy children.

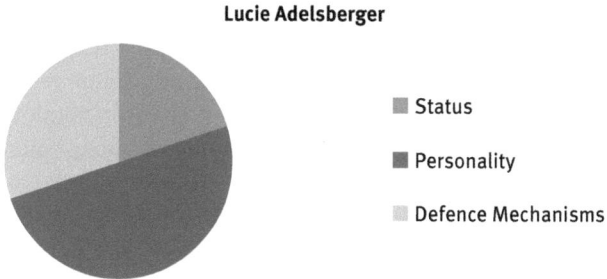

Fig. 31: Survival primarily dependent upon Personal Traits and to a lessor extent Defence Mechanisms.

Maximilian Samuel

Samuel took advantage of his status as a colleague of SS doctors to aid in his survival. His main defence mechanisms were rationalization and denial. He believed that by collaborating with the SS he was saving his own life and that of his daughter. His personal characteristics included resilience, determination and cunning.

Maximilian Samuel

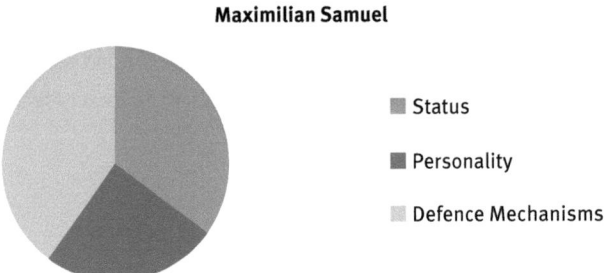

- Status
- Personality
- Defence Mechanisms

Fig. 32: Samuel survived until he was executed by taking advantage of his Status and by Defence Mechanisms.

In her article *Explanations for Survival by Jewish Survivors of the Holocaust* (n.d.), Jennie Goldenberg examines the reasons for survival according to survivors of the Holocaust. Goldenberg examines the role of internal and external attributions. She cites internal attributions such as intelligence and skill, facility with languages or being an intentional doer selecting, constructing and regulating one's own activity to realize certain outcomes. Goldenberg argues:

> Decision-making abilities and perseverance are internal attributions survivors cite which can be placed under the larger category of agency. Self-efficacy, or belief in oneself and one's abilities, is a related concept. (Goldenberg, n.d.)

According to Goldenberg external attributions include factors beyond the survivor's control such as help from others and luck, faith or fate. She contends that external attributions are personal characteristics that do not imply personal control; they just 'are', such as physical appearance and health. Goldenberg questions Frankl's emphasis on the meaning in life as a determining attribution to survival. She maintains that given the suffering in the hell of the camps and ghettos, survival was more dependent on resilience. Goldenberg's construct of survival has similarities with the model I have proposed here but there are significant differences. The cohort examined here represents Jewish prisoners of Auschwitz, a death camp where the SS had the goal of murdering every Jew that entered the camp, whereas Goldenberg's sample included survivors of ghettos, other camps and people who survived in hiding. Her presentation does not distinguish between survivors of ghettoes or camps and does not provide information concerning time incarcerated or in hiding, even though the experience of being in an extermination camp is vastly different from being in hiding. Where a survivor was an inmate of a camp, she provides no information on the type of work he or she performed. Her research presents the explanations survivors gave for their survival, and concentrates on what she classifies as internal attributions, such as the will to live, personal characteristics and agency, and external attributions, such as help from others, God, miracles and luck. The construct presented in this current study is more structured and relies on an in-depth examination of memoirs, oral testimonies and interviews of Jewish doctor survivors and their families. Goldenberg's study appears to have been conducted more along the lines of a questionnaire. Survivors' responses to Goldenberg's question of how they survived included luck (37 out of 154), God (29 out of 154) and miracles (24 out of 154). Thus more emphasis was placed on external attributions than on personal strengths and activities. Despite their responses, Goldenberg concedes that survival depends on more than luck and God.

The construct I have presented here can be extrapolated to other survivors of Auschwitz. As I have argued, surviving Auschwitz over a relatively long period was impossible without both internal strengths and external privileges. Such external privileges were also available to other prisoners, such as clerks, cooks, Kapos, block elders and workers in Kanada, who enjoyed 'prominent' status and benefitted accordingly. Other Jewish doctor survivors, such as Nyiszli, Cohen, Epstein, Grunwald, Wolken, Beijlin, Imrene, Fleck and Fejkiel, were also privileged prisoners, some more than others. Due to their status and importance to the SS, their basic needs were met. To survive they needed to be mentally hardy and resilient, amongst other traits, and to have found a meaning in life. Upon examination each of these doctors was involved in or committed to a cause or an activity that gave him or her meaning in life. For Epstein it was scientific research, for Cohen the care of the mentally ill, for Wolken the obsessive keeping of records, for Fleck and Fejkiel research, for Grunwald the treatment of patients and his close relationship with and care of his son, and for Nyiszli it was commitment to his work with Mengele and the Sonderkommandos.

Non-medical survivors

Two non-medical prisoners of Auschwitz who were interviewed also relied on status, personal traits and defence mechanisms to survive: Kalman Bar On, who survived ten months of hell after becoming a Mengele twins with his sister, and

Zippi Tichauer, who was in Auschwitz from 28 March 1942 for almost three years. The following brief profiles of Kalman and Zippy demonstrate that the model for survival also applied to non-medical prisoners.

Kalman Bar On

Kalman[77] was a thirteen-year-old boy when he entered Auschwitz. He arrived dressed in his best clothes thinking he and his family were going to be resettled and perhaps start a new life. Instead he entered a world of loneliness, fear, brutality, filth, degradation and death. Yet he survived.

Kalman and his twin sister Judit were born on 30 May 1930 in Ilok, Hungary. Their father died when the twins were only two years old leaving their mother Tova to raise Kalman and his four siblings. Two of the brothers, Joseph and Moses, died of illness during their early years but Kalman's mother struggled on, displaying resilience and discipline in coping with what Kalman describes as a life 'on the wrong side of an average existence.' The family was adopted by his paternal grandfather Braun, who provided for them both materially and by ensuring that the children received a traditional orthodox upbringing. He was an honest, conservative man, who insisted that life was guided by the Talmud. Consequently, the twins were sent to a Jewish primary school. Kalman received very strict religious schooling all the way through to high school. Under the guidance of his grandfather, he would study the Talmud upon rising early in the morning and before going to bed at night. He had a happy life as a young boy despite the hardship and felt secure and protected

However, like many Jews in Hungary, the Braun family was subject to abuse and the uncertainty and prejudices of antisemitism. Kalman remembers being escorted to school by his grandfather, who would position the young boy between him and the wall so that any stones thrown at them would not hit Kalman. Thus antisemitism was well embedded into the Hungarian psyche and culture long before Hitler came to power in Germany and eventually in Hungary.

Sunday 19 March 1944 would change life forever for Kalman. His family, including his grandfather, were forced into the ghetto and eventually sent to Auschwitz. Only he and his twin sister would survive; his grandfather was murdered in the gas chambers on arrival in Auschwitz; his mother perished on the death march.

The train journey to Auschwitz was similar to that endured by over one million Jews from all over German-occupied Europe. Once at Auschwitz, the family was

---

77 The author conducted a series of interviews with Mr Bar On during 2011 in Tel-Aviv.

subject to the same procedures that met all newcomers to the death camp: 'Raus! Raus! Schnell! Schnell!' All of this experienced in darkness, with shouting, dogs barking, whips cracking, shots ringing out, people in striped pyjama-type clothing trying to direct the new arrivals. Kalman was herded into the same section as his mother and sister but once the children were identified as twins, they were directed to the KB camp for twins. Kalman was directed to the block for male twins, dwarves and gypsy children while his sister was sent to the female block. Both became exclusive members of the group known as the 'Mengele twins', guinea pigs in Mengele's medical experiments to create a superior German race. As a result he became a privileged prisoner. The basic physical needs of the twins and dwarves were sufficiently met to keep them alive. At least until they had fulfilled their purpose; after that most were murdered.

One of the most valued and life-saving graces for Kalman was his close friendship with Ludovivz Feld, a dwarf. Due to his small stature and lack of strength, Ludovivz needed a strong young boy to fight for him at meal times to get him bread and sausage. Kalman in turn profited from Ludovivz's wisdom and cunning on how to survive in such a hostile world. Another fortunate occurrence for Kalman was being selected to work in the guards' quarters cleaning the floors, polishing their shoes and, best of all, cleaning their eating utensils after meals, along with another young boy, Lipot Lowy, known as 'Lippa'. Not only were the two boys protected from the harsh elements, excused from roll calls and protected from severe punishment, they were blessed with access to the leftovers of the guards. Kalman would take his share to divide it between Ludovivz and his sister and his mother, who were living in the women's experimental block.

Three times a month, Kalman was brought into the military leaders' block to be examined. The examination would take place in the presence of a Jewish doctor called Epstein, Mengele, and a French Jewess, who Kalman believed was a physiotherapist or social worker of some sort, and usually two members of the SS. While Epstein was kind and gentle, the French woman was sterner and demanding. Before inspection the children had to ensure they were clean and their clothes were as free of lice as was possible. Kalman describes the atmosphere as one of fear and terror. They had no certainty whether they would survive the examination as they knew that on a whim, Mengele could have them subjected to some type of surgery or medical procedure. Kalman recalled that although he could remove the dirt and lice, he could never shed the unbearable feelings of terror and fear. Nevertheless, in a perverse kind of way, Kalman was one of the luckier children. He recalls a set of twins one of whom had a good singing voice. Mengele decided to operate on the voice box of each child and only one survived the ordeal. The purpose of this operation was not apparent to anyone but Mengele. Despite being treated a little better than the other prisoners, prison life was very harsh for Kalman and the other 'Mengele children'. At the end of each day, Kalman would race back to his block to eat and then climb into his bunk and snuggle into the protective sheltering arms of Ludovivz.

Kalman believes both his heritage and the early discipline and religious teachings imparted by his paternal grandfather provided him with the strength and resilience to survive: the strength to wrestle with what could be overcome and the good sense to hide, bend or run from things that could not. He never felt sorry for himself but seemed to have had the ability to accept his situation without surrendering to it, confirming Frankl's observation that 'everything can be taken from a man but one thing: the last of human freedoms – to choose one's attitude in any given circumstances, to choose one's own way' (Frankl, 1959, 86).

Kalman did not have an abundance of food but he had enough to survive. The opportunity to obtain additional to provide for his family and protect his friends became a commitment and a responsibility that in turn protected him from the culture of the camp. His socialization in his early life gave him strength and self-esteem. While he never felt secure and lived in fear and a state of anxiety, he had experienced hatred of Jews and discrimination and could cope to an extent. He did not have to attend roll calls and was not subject to daily selections. The greatest gift he received was friendship and a close relationship with Ludovivz and Lippa. He was resilient and determined. He was vigilant to danger and accepted that he was in a vicious uncontrollable situation and that he needed to take action to protect himself, his family and friends. The commitment to his sister, mother and friends by providing extra food was his priority. He understood that keeping on side with the SS would enable him to get further privileges and that this gave him the best chance of surviving.

Kalman entered Auschwitz in early July 1944. He was only a young boy but he had the personal traits, some privileges and a reason and will to live. He survived, as did his sister. Their mother died during the death march. After eventually migrating to Israel, Kalman married and became a father; he still leads a meaningful life. He has kept the memory of the Holocaust alive by telling his story.

Tichauer Helen 'Zippi'

Helen Tichauer[78], known as Zippy, arrived in Auschwitz on 28 March 1942. She was imprisoned in the camp for three years and survived. This was an

---

[78] The author conducted a series of interviews with Ms Tichauer during 2010 and 2011 in New York and by phone.

extraordinary achievement. What separated her from the majority of prisoners who died or were executed? Closer examination of Zippi's life and experience show that her survival over a long period fits the model presented. According to Professor Konrad Kwiet, who interviewed Zippi, she spent her childhood and teens in the comfortable environment of a caring Jewish home. She grew up in a modern Jewish household where religious observance was expected, education was encouraged and social service was natural. Her mother died when she was only six years old and she and her brother lived with her maternal grandmother. With her grandmother's encouragement Zippi became an avid reader. German was her mother tongue, but she lived in a multinational and multilingual environment and attended classes in French and Hebrew. She was highly successful at school and at college, where she was accepted to study design. This was a man's profession at the time but Zippy was not deterred.

Arriving at Auschwitz Zippi experienced the humiliating and brutal processing to which all prisoners were subject and was assigned to the Stammlager Birkenau. She was initially assigned to hard labour but was injured in an accident and thereafter assigned to the Häftlingsschreibstube, the prisoner office, as a scribe/designer. This provided her with better conditions and protected her from much of the misery suffered by other prisoners. The SS became aware of Zippi's qualifications as a designer and she was given the task of creating a system to mark and identify prisoners. This assignment was to last the duration of her captivity. This assignment gave her the status of a 'prominent' that gave her privileges such as more food, better clothing and cleaner accommodation, better sanitary conditions and the respect of the Nazis. She had access to all camps without supervision and at times was allowed outside the camps to visit outlying villages and towns and for picnics.

In interviews with Kwiet and later with myself she presented as a resilient, assertive even stubborn person who was inventive and anticipatory. In addition to speaking German, French and Hebrew, she learned Polish, Russian and Yiddish in Auschwitz, and her language skills became a lifesaver: They helped her foster relationships with the SS, the Kapos and fellow prisoners. Zippi obviously had a strong will to live but she also found meaning in life while she was in Auschwitz. Her commitment to her work was a defence mechanism and according to Vaillant's model would be an example of sublimation, the ability to become immersed in a project. That Zippi was committed to excellence impressed the SS and she was given the opportunity to become involved in other meaningful projects. She also played in the camp orchestra, which gave her further interests. To some extent, Zippi also had luck: being assigned to the Häftlings-schreibstube, allowed her skills as a designer to come to the attention of the SS.

In the case of Zippi it is contended that all three factors or components of the model co-existed for survival. She could not have survived Auschwitz for three years without the better conditions that came with being a 'privileged' or 'prominent' prisoner. She had resilience, determination and self-esteem, arguably as a result of her socialization as a young person. Finally, she became immersed in a project, design and architecture, which lasted from 1942 to 1945.

Zippy undertook the death march and first arrived at Ravensbrück then Malchow, a sub camp of Ravensbrück. This camp was liberated by the Russians in May, 1945. After a long journey home to Bratislava she found antisemitism was unbearable and she went to a DP camp (displace camp) in Central Europe. In Feldafing she met and married Erwin Tichauer. They secured papers to leave Europe and began a nomadic but highly successful life in several countries, including Australia, Chile, Indonesia and finally the United States. Zippy throughout continued as a freelance graphic designer and Erwin worked for the United Nations and entered academia becoming an eminent scholar.

Surviving Auschwitz was complicated and multifaceted. It was not due to a single factor unless one considered a scenario in which the camp was used, as a transit station for a prisoner(s) such as was the case of Viktor Frankl. Although respecting those who believed in miracles, happenance and or God, for a prisoner to survive for a relative long period, such as four or six months and longer, an amalgam of personal traits, protective techniques and privileges were essential. Each of the survivors studied, revealed varying degrees of dependence on each of the components of survival. The doctors were at the epicentre of the evil and suffering that was visited upon the Jewish population. First they suffered similar fear and anxiety of any human under a death sentence. Second arguably more than any prisoner they were witness to death and suffering almost every minute of every day and probably the most tragic they were forced to abandon their professional code of ethics and personal morals and do harm to patients and were unable to protect them. Third, on occasions they were unwillingly involved in prisoners' executions. To overcome these physical, psychological, emotional and ethical challenges and survive required the doctor to rise almost beyond human endurance. They each unconsciously and consciously arrived at the same destination using the same map but followed a slightly different path.

Part VI: **Evaluation of Sources**

Historians often insist that they come to their research with a tabula rasa, that they judge each situation on its merits and do not let other matters shape their perceptions. In fact, no matter how much they may deny it, their personal experiences constitute facets on the prism through which their view of past events is refracted. For the sake of her readers and herself, a historian must acknowledge their presence and try to ensure that they clarify, rather than cloud, her understanding

Lipstadt (2011)

To complete this work, I have relied principally on memoirs, and witness testimonies and statements. Normally archives and historiography are the main source of research. However, most of the documents including medical reports, charts, details of medications and medical supplies and death books[79] were destroyed prior to and during the Nazis' flight from the camp in 1945. Many of the documents and reports that have survived are false (Shelley 1986). Details of prisoner histories in the camp are limited, particularly in relation to Jewish doctors. In the case of the Jewish doctors whose biographies are presented here, archival evidence of their arrival and life in Auschwitz is almost non-existent. The only official record of Sima Vaisman's imprisonment is her listing on a transport train from Drancy. No records of Giselle Perl's history in Auschwitz exist. Only memoirs and survivor testimonials verify her work.

The story could not be told without the published and unpublished memoirs of survivor doctors. In examining the memoirs as a source, it must be noted that: First, the sameness of the descriptions of conditions and the culture of evil and inhumanity gives legitimacy to their stories of life in the camp. Second, a difference in style and language between genders becomes obvious. Third, questions of accuracy and reliability arise. Finally, the period the memoirs were written – some immediately after the war, others thirty to fifty years later – is reflected in the emotion felt and language used. The memoirs are emotional and confronting. Langer argues, 'the impossibility ... lies not in the reality but in our difficulty in perceiving it as reality' (Langer 1991, 40). All the reader or scholar can do is to acknowledge the suffering and conditions but under no circumstances can they truly comprehend. The reader can, however, understand the survivor having feelings of anger, despair, helplessness and fear.

The autobiographies are in most cases articulate and provide the reader with descriptions of epic events and profoundly disturbing scenes. For most survivors they are an attempt to express feelings of frustration and despair that words cannot convey. Philosopher and French art historian Georges Didi-Huberman,

---

[79] Death books contained the names of prisoners who died and the causes of death. In most cases causes of death were fabricated.

https://doi.org/10.1515/9783110598216-017

arguably one of the most important art theorists, contends that feelings and emotions cannot be felt despite efforts to capture them through words, poetry and sketches and paintings. Thus the observer may read the words but they are impossible to comprehend. It is beyond the observer to understand the degree of fear, hopelessness, suffering and utter helplessness that gripped the prisoner. That is one of the reasons many survivors refused to talk of their experiences. They could not put their experiences into words and those who did, could not convey the emotion or feelings. Many survivors do not want to, or find it difficult, to revive their experiences and the suffering. Heda Kovály recalls her reluctance to record her memories of the Holocaust:

> I do not want to write. I do not want to remember. My memories are not simple recollections. They are a return to the bottom of the abyss; I have to gather up the shattered bones that have lain still for so long, climb back over the crags and tumble in once more. Only this time I have to do it deliberately, in slow motion, noticing and examining each wound, each bruise on the way, most of all the ones of which I was least conscious in my headlong fall. But I know I have to do it. My future stands aside, waiting until I find meaning in all that has been. I feel as if I had to overcome some almost physical obstacle and feel drained, breathless from the effort. (Kovály & Kohák 1973)

Is Kovály's reluctance the desire to put the past behind her and try to lead a normal life? Langer argues that memory imprisons the consciousness, therefore recounting the story should be liberating. As long as memory is in control, the survivor or one who has been traumatised, cannot escape the nightmare. Nietzsche (1980), felt that, 'without forgetting it is impossible to live at all'. In answer to Nietzsche: It may be impossible to forget experiences of indescribable evil, which is why many survivors find it difficult to lead a normal life. Few survivors can express the emotion of the victims as succinctly as Eli Wiesel or Jean Améry. And yet, Wiesel (2006) confessed his impotence in trying to express himself as a witness, of watching helplessly as language became an obstacle to expression, knowing that it would be necessary to invent a new language. The words he used or offered seemed to him 'meagre, pale, lifeless.' Despite his feelings of inadequacy, he provides a vivid glimpse of the deprivation and horror. His description of the horrendous journey to Auschwitz is one that draws the observer into a world of inhumanity and its consequences:

> Was there a way to describe the last journey in sealed cattle cars, the last voyage toward the unknown? Or the discovery of a demented and glacial universe where to be inhuman was to be human, where disciplined, educated men in uniform came to kill and innocent children and weary old men came to die? Or the countless separations on a single fiery night, the tearing apart of whole families, entire communities? Or, incredibly, the vanishing of a beautiful, well-behaved little Jewish girl with golden hair and a sad smile, murdered with

her mother the very night of their arrival? How was one to speak of them without trembling and a heart broken for all eternity? (Améry 1986)

Wiesel describes exactly what he perceived succinctly, yet in his eyes he has failed to convey what the victims feel such that the observer, the outsider, could ever understand the suffering and terror. He resigns himself to the fact that, 'only those who experienced Auschwitz know what it was. Others will never know' (Wiesel 2006). Améry feels the same inadequacy when retelling his experience of being tortured:

> It would be totally senseless to try and describe here the pain that was inflicted on me ... Qualities of feeling are as incomparable as they indescribable. They mark the limit of the capacity of language to communicate. In the bunker there hung from the vaulted ceiling a chain that above ran into a roll. At its bottom end it bore a heavy, broadly curved iron hook ... The hook gripped into the shackle that held my hands together behind my back. Then I was raised with the chain until I was hung about a meter over the floor ... All your life is gathered in a single, limited area of the body, the shoulder joints and it does not react; for it exhausts itself completely in the expenditure of energy ... And now there was a crackling and splintering in my shoulders that my body has not forgotten until this hour ... My own body weight caused luxation; I fell into a void and now hung by my dislocated arms, which had been torn high from behind and were now twisted over my head. Torture, from Latin torquere, to twist ... At the same time, the blows from the horsewhip showered down on my body and some of them sliced cleanly through the light summer trousers that I was wearing on this twenty-third of July 1943. (Améry, 1986, 32)

Langer discusses survivor Irene W, who upon returning home after liberation, tried to tell people what happened to her family:

> She remembers thinking that 'My family were killed' was totally inadequate because 'killed,' she says, was a word used for 'ordinary' forms of dying. But to say matter-of-factly that, 'My mother and brother and two sisters were gassed' as soon as they arrived at Auschwitz seemed equally unsatisfactory, because plain factuality could not convey the enormity of the event. (Langer 1991, 61)

Apparently Irene W was especially reluctant to reduce her family's fate to just a statistic. Langer argues there are limits to the memory's ability to recreate the past such that the reader understands. He refers to the testimony of E. Chaim, a survivor of Sobibor, who felt that an essential part of his story was lost in the retelling:

> It is just impossible. The only one who has lived it through know [sic] what really happened. Because the feelings that are involved with this story, they are not the same. You cannot – feelings you can bring, to a certain degree – tell what it is. You cannot tell how I felt when I found the clothes of my brother, for example [while sorting the garments of those who

had been gassed]. Now if you asked what I had been thinking about, I wasn't thinking at all. I was horrified ... But I can tell the story and it sounds – well, [like] another story. But it is more than another story. It is more some feeling what you cannot bring out, you know. (Langer 1991, 62)

Inarguably Chaim is speaking for many survivors either when they attempt to write of their experiences or speak of their life in Auschwitz or any of the camps. They fear their story would be seen as a fabrication, as Langer observes:

It is not surprising to hear witnesses in oral testimonies confess that sometimes they do not believe their own stories. Their effort to recapture through memory what, because of the impossibility of its content, has already (for us) fallen outside memory, risks estranging the audience they seek to inform. (Langer 1991, 40)

According to Delbo, 'Today, I am no longer sure that what I have written is true, but I am sure that it happened' (Delbo 1986, 72).

An examination of the memoirs reveals a gender difference in both language and expression. Those written by female doctors are in most cases more descriptive and emotional. They provide vivid descriptions of conditions and feelings that reveal unimaginable treatment of humans. Paradoxically they focus on both the order and chaos of life in the camp. Order is described in the intolerable roll calls that had to be accurate, the daily inspections of blocks, selections that followed a specific ritual, and the fanatical obsession to keep records and documentation. There is even order in the falsification of medical documents. They describe the chaos of the indescribably inhumane conditions, the uncontrolled epidemics, horrific sanitary conditions, the scenes of panic and hysteria when prisoners and patients were loaded onto trucks destined for the gas chambers or the fire pits, the random beatings resulting in death and the chaos before the evacuation and dreaded death march.[80]

The memoirs of the men mostly concentrate on their own feelings and survival. Descriptions of camp conditions are addressed but in more detached terms. A disproportionate number of male doctors were involved in experimental work. While living in constant fear for their life, they were not as exposed to the shocking conditions that other prisoners endured in Birkenau or the labour camps. An example of the stark difference between the writings of the genders is

---

80 The Death March refers to the forced marches by the inmates of the camps, this case Auschwitz, under guard after the evacuation of the camp. The SS euphemistically called the death marches *Evakuierung* (evacuation). Many thousands of prisoners died from exhaustion, froze to death or were executed during the long journey. The SS moved the prisoners from one camp to another in an effort to continue to exploit their labor.

demonstrated when Nyiszli describes the pyres into which Jews were thrown after being shot, some still alive. Nyiszli shows very little emotion:

> The pyre was a ditch, 50 metres long, 6 metres wide and 3 metres deep, containing hundreds of burning bodies. Each pyre was surrounded by SS-men holding special six-millimetre guns for shooting in the back of the head ... even the crack of the pistol was drowned out by the ghastly screams of dying people. The bullet fired from a small-calibre pistol was usually insufficient to kill the victim, who was then cast into the inferno still alive. (Nyiszli 1993, 65)

Adelsberger expresses far more emotion in describing the same event:

> The inside walls of our block were lit up with the reflection of the blaze. And when we got up and crept out the back doors of the block that faced the crematorium opposite and looked toward the second one, I saw the flames of the open fire next to it and watched as they tossed the dead (and sometimes not quite dead) bodies of children onto it. I heard their screams, saw how the fire lapped at their tender bodies. No metamorphosis of my being, regardless of whether in this life or the next, will ever expunge this horror from my soul. (Adelsberger 1969, 85)

Adelsberger focuses on the horror of the children being murdered and discarded as if they were meat or rubbish while Nyiszli concentrates on the logistics and structure. The memoirs identify the female doctors as nurturers and comforters and this is reflected in their prose and language. Although memoirs and testimonies provide a rich cache of accounts of life in Auschwitz they also raise important questions. What role do testimonies play in substantiating facts? What insights do they provide? Are testimonies or memoirs written immediately after the war more authentic and accurate than those recorded thirty to forty years after the event? Are the immediate testimonies clouded by trauma and raw emotions? Are later narratives coloured by collective memory formed by society, the media, Holocaust survivor social groups and the subsequent life of the individual after the Holocaust? (Ofer 2008, 532) What is to be made of memoirs and testimonies that are inaccurate or questionable? Richard Seaver in his introduction to Nyiszli's memoir states, 'inevitably and inexorably, history reduces the personal to the impersonal subsumes the individual into the collective, renders the immediate remote' (Nyiszli 1993, 5). Memoirs and testimonies by survivors are essential personal accounts of the Holocaust that preserve the immediacy of what happened and that keep their memories alive and accessible. Survivors need to tell their stories even if it is impossible for us to understand the full extent of their suffering or the horror of what transpired. Memory can be an accurate story of what happened or was said, or it can be distorted be it by emotions, time, mental capacity and age. My approach has been to make what I believe is a critical but fair examination of memoirs and testimonies.

Reading a memoir or listening to a testimony once is not enough. To authenticate the conditions or cruelty of the camps it is necessary to read and analyse the memoirs a number of times. I accept there will be discrepancies and poor memory particularly as age and time advances or as a result of loss and trauma. Memoirs written from the early 1980s to the present appear to be less detailed, less emotional and more circumspect than those written earlier. Perl and Vaisman wrote their memoirs immediately after liberation and their emotions of anger, hate and revenge spill almost from every page. Micheels, who wrote his memoirs in the late 1980s, showed less rage and hatred towards the Nazis and even had positive words to say about SS Dr Hans Münch.[81] Astonishingly Micheels claimed 'there were actually times without acute stress when I found myself musing that ... my life was not so impossible' (Micheels 1989, 193).

For the influence of the media there is no better example than that of Mengele, who somehow managed to slip under the radar and to avoid notoriety until after 1960. From that period onwards, many survivors claim to have encountered Mengele at the time of arriving at Auschwitz or during their hospitalization whilst in the camp. On some days up to six thousand Jews arrived in Auschwitz making it very difficult if not impossible for Mengele to be present at every arrival. From the 1970s onwards Mengele has appeared in many texts detailing his role at Auschwitz, rightly demonizing him for his cruel and ruthless actions. However, this wide publicity and subsequent infamy appears to have given licence for his name to appear in almost every testimony and memoir.

Christopher Browning refers to testimonies by Starachowice survivors, including those who were children at the time, whose transport entered Birkenau without the normal decimating selection on the ramp. Browning claims the witness statements are repetitive in themselves and repeat what others have said.

> Yet a number of testimonies nonetheless relate that the transport was subjected to selection on the ramp, with none other than the notorious Dr Josef Mengele himself directing people to the right and the left ... both the memories of the majority concerning the very atypical entry into Birkenau (which could hardly have been invented and shared by so many if it had not happened) and the very survival of children who lived to testify because of that atypical entry provide convincing evidence that there was no such Mengele-led selection on the ramp immediately following arrival in Birkenau, the firmly held belief of other survivors notwithstanding. (Browning 2010, 11)

Browning (2010) argues that 'the historian should concede that serious problems confront the use of such eyewitness accounts as a source'. He goes on to say,

---

81 Dr Hans Münch was a SS doctor at Auschwitz from 1943 to 1945. He was the only person acquitted at the War Crimes trials in Kraków.

The situation is even more problematic in the case of writing Holocaust history, because of the traumatic experiences of the witnesses, the understandable urge to treat less critically the testimony of those who have suffered so greatly and widespread popular representation that has created iconic images and tropes that have been incorporated into subsequent memory. (Browning 2010, 12)

Having examined the problems of later testimonies, Browning argues that there is a foundation upon which reliable testimonies are built:

What emerges from a critical mass of testimony …is a core memory that has remained basically stable despite the passage of time and the geographical dispersion of the survivor communities. With such a core memory, some reasonable judgments about plausibility can be made about various individual memories based on the overall credibility of the survivor's testimony, the vividness and detail of the particular events being recalled, the absence of contradiction with other plausible narratives and – to be honest – the highly subjective intuition of the individual historian that gradually develops from prolonged immersion in the materials. (Browning 2010, 12)

Browning is correct, for it is only through examining many memoirs and oral testimonies that a clear picture evolves which either substantiates the event or conditions or provides grounds to dismiss the claims. By contrast, the same atmosphere and emotions during selections of both patient and prisoner doctor described repeatedly may or may not be testimony to their authenticity. Scholar Lucy Dawidowicz does not attach much authority to testimonies:

The transcribed testimonies I have examined have been full of errors in dates, names of participants and places and there are evident misunderstandings of the events themselves. (Dawidowicz 1981, 177)

After extensive examination the accuracy and reliability of some sections of particular memoirs can be questioned. While every memoir arguably has some questionable recollections, there are glaring omissions and contradictions in the Jewish doctors' memoirs that must be noted. The memoirs of Perl and Lengyel indicate discrepancy in respect to the same event. Olga Lengyel (1995) states she accompanied a friend P when P was ordered to perform an abortion on Irma Grese, a much-feared female guard in Birkenau. Lengyel states that Grese drew a gun on P in the infirmary and ordered her to go to Grese's apartment. Lengyel states P asked her to be her nurse. Perl in her memoirs describes the scene, the fear of being sent to the gas and also the fact that Grese had a gun under her pillow. Perl does not mention the scene in the infirmary or Lengyel's presence in her description of the abortion.

Further, Perl in her memoir states that her son Imre went to Auschwitz with her and the family. From both her memoir and a film of her life after the Holocaust,

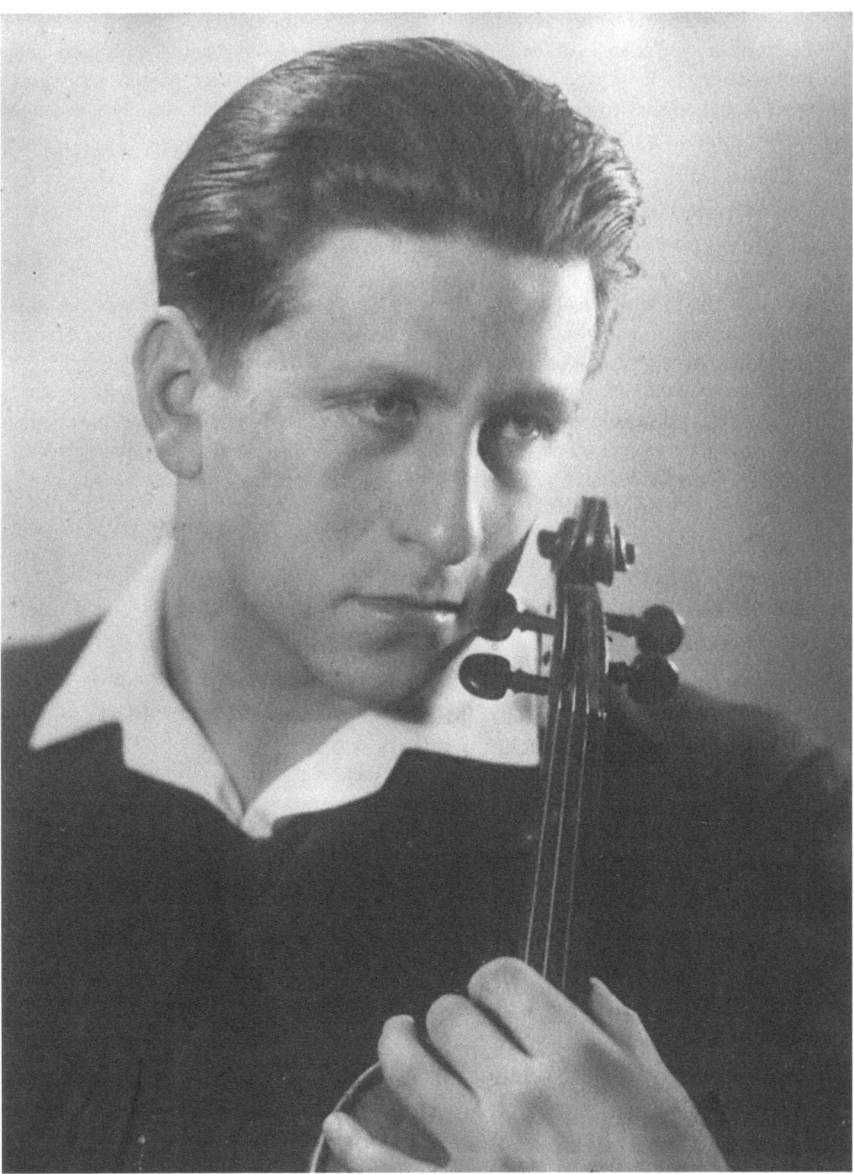

Fig. 33: Imre Aged 20 before the War probably 1940.
(Courtesy Ella Krause, daughter and Giora Kraus, grandson of Dr Perl)

Imre is portrayed as a twelve year or fourteen-year-old boy. Yet from photographs of Imre prior to the war, he appears to be in his early twenties. According to Ella, Perl's daughter, Imre did not go to Auschwitz but to a labour camp where he was beaten to death. Strangely, Perl at no point mentions her daughter Ella in her memoirs or on film. According to Ella, her mothers' story of the family adopting a Christian girl was incorrect. The exclusion of Ella, who I met and interviewed in Haifa with her son Giora, and the fate of Imre, raise the question of accuracy and creditability.

The biography of Brewda, which portrays her as a caring, loyal and selfless person, is brought into question when we consider that her prisoner colleague, Ima Spanjaard, who also worked in Block 10, describes her as someone who lived very well in the camp while her patients were dying from starvation and dysentery (Shelley 1991, 51). There is no other evidence accusing Brewda of being selfish or acting against the interests of the prisoners; other witnesses described her as a caring, selfless doctor. Numerous memoirs describe scenes of sexual activity in the latrines that give the impression of rampant sexual activity. Yet survivors maintained that sexual desire and urges were the first to go 'many of us young men ceased to have any sexual feelings whatever ... during all the time we were in Treblinka and for long afterwards, we were men in name only' (Sereny 2000, 237).

Frankl recalls a prisoner of Auschwitz who 'even in his dreams ... did not seem to concern himself with sex' (Frankl 1959). The exhaustion and emaciation of prisoners and the lack of food and vitamins destroyed sexual drive and caused sexual dysfunction. Sex between prisoners was forbidden so they were taking a risk of punishment if caught. However, sex must have been happening since female prisoners did fall pregnant. A memoir that has recently been subject to close examination is that of Frankl's' life during the Holocaust. With the exception of the latest edition of *Man's Search for Meaning,* one has the distinct impression that he was a prisoner in Auschwitz for a relatively long period. This is false. Frankl spent two to three days in Auschwitz before he was sent to Kaufering III, one of many satellite camps of Dachau, in which he was incarcerated for approximately five months. Nevertheless, Améry wrote, 'The Viennese doctor Dr Viktor Frankl ... was for years a ditch digger in Auschwitz-Monowitz' (Améry 1986, 3). Before Auschwitz, Frankl and his family were sent to Theresienstadt where they were prisoners for two years. It was both a ghetto and concentration camp. Frankl does not mention Theresienstadt. A number of discrepancies become apparent that indicate Frankl was not in Auschwitz for as long a period as he infers. Frankl arrived at Auschwitz in early October and recalls that 'for days we were unable to wash, even partially, because of frozen water pipes' (Frankl 1959, 14). In October do temperatures fall to levels that would cause water pipes to freeze? He claims 'we had to wear the same shirts for half the year.' He comments that 'after a few months' stay in the camp, we could not walk up those steps'. While Frankl may have had these experiences, it is unlikely that they occurred during his brief stay in Auschwitz. The reader also gains the impression that Frankl's' logotherapy model was created in the camps based on his experiences and those of the prisoners. According to Timothy Pytell, Frankl developed and formalized his model in the early 1930s 'and, according to Pytell (2000), 'his prescription for youths in distress was a call for them to find a mission' or meaning in life. Pytell argues,

> Frankl's logotherapy is not simply a product of his (embellished) concentration camp experiences, but is actually rooted in a rejection of Freudian materialism in the early 1920s and problemised (sic) by his attempt to accommodate an organization of German psychotherapists that was sponsored by the Nazi regime. (Pytell 2000, 281)

There is no doubt Frankl experienced monstrous conditions, hardship and brutality in the ghettos and concentration and labour camps. One would think, however, that Frankl's' experience in Theresienstadt, of brutality, sickness, starvation and death followed by similar conditions in the labour camps of Dachau would provide him with sufficient insight and material to develop further and reinforce logotherapy and the theory of the meaning in life. Why he persisted in representing his suffering and ordeals as taking place in Auschwitz is not known. He claims, 'facts will be significant only as far as they are part of a man's experience' (Frankl 1959, 5). But if the facts are based on deception or embellished, how can they be part of one's experience? Unfortunately, Frankl is no longer alive to debate the issues Pytell has brought to the table of Holocaust testimony and memoirs.

It is not the intention here to judge or devalue the content of the memoirs or the memories and recollections of the authors. Memoirs, written and oral, of Holocaust survivors must be respected and accepted as genuine interpretations of what they believed took place in Auschwitz and all camps. However, in researching and writing history it is the responsibility of the historian to constructively and critically examine events that took place. Where a memoir has inconsistencies or appears to be embellished, does it throw a shadow over the entire memoir or over memoirs as a source? Do testimonies need to be completely accurate? Why should it throw doubt on all memoirs when one prisoner doctor tells of starting the daily clinic at 4 am when another reports the clinics began at 7 am? They are stories filled with trauma and emotions yet they are accurate and reliable in the sense that they represent collective memories that legitimize and confirm the whole picture.

When one survivor's account of an event or circumstance is repeated in exactly the same by dozens of other survivors, men and women in different camps, from different nations and cultures, then one comes to trust the validity of such reports and even to question departures from the general view (Des Pres, 1976, 11). According to Philip Friedman (1980, 556), 'the first reaction of the survivors after their liberation was a passionate desire to dramatize the impact of the past experience' proposing there was a spirit of martyrology emanating from literature on the Holocaust that prevented a clear-cut view from an historical perspective. Even so, it is important to accept there will be inconsistencies and inaccuracies when examining and analysing memoirs. In saying that, it is also necessary for the researcher and reader not to necessarily accept what is on the surface, but to look deeper and decide upon the legitimacy and worth of the recollections and accounts. This particularly applies to different descriptions and accounts of the same event. It can be argued that it is natural for people to distort or embellish events that occurred both for their own and for the benefit of their audience.

One of the pillars of the construct explaining how Jewish doctors survived consists of defence mechanisms and coping skills that are described and discussed in psychological and psychosocial literature. I have relied upon a comprehensive range of authoritative works by Sigmund and Anna Freud, George Eman Vaillant, Ervin Staub, Jesse Prinz, Robert Jay Lifton, Susan B. Fine and survivors such as, psychiatrists Elie Cohen, Viktor Frankl and Bruno Bettelheim. Freud's theory of ego defence mechanisms provides answers to how prisoners faced with adversity cope with their changed circumstances. Vaillant presents a model of defence mechanisms that explains the different strategies, conscious or unconscious, which assist the subject to overcome adversity or cope with the circumstances presented. Fine presents a paper on resilience and adaptability that fits well with this study while Prinz has studied the question of the impact of nature and nurture on human behaviour. Prinz argues socialization has the dominant role in moulding character and resilience and his argument is embraced in this work. In this study emphasis has been placed on Vaillant's theory of defence mechanisms.

I have briefly treated the contribution of historical narrative. This source has contributed much to our knowledge of the history of the Holocaust from the viewpoint of the perpetrator, victim and bystander. Unfortunately, there are pockets of Holocaust history that have not been thoroughly researched; these include the life, work and survival of Jewish doctors in the camps. The work of Jay Lifton, Nadav, Herman Langbein, Ruth Jolanda Weinberger, Laurence Rees, Ley and Volume IV Auschwitz by Auschwitz-Birkenau State Museum have contributed to a limited extent to the body of knowledge of the efforts of Jewish doctors. Jay Lifton has concentrated on the psychological interpretation of the Third Reich from a medical perspective. He has provided three chapters on the life of prisoner doctors in Auschwitz addressing such subjects as the struggle to heal, to fight against the lure of collaboration and to cope with selections. He provides insight into the terrible dilemmas faced by every prisoner doctor including Jewish doctors. His work is ground-breaking in the sense that it provides an answer to the question of how ordinary people, in this case SS doctors, can commit evil through the concepts of 'doubling,' and 'numbing'. Lifton is the only historian who has devoted a number of chapters to prisoner doctors in the Holocaust. But here again it is not solely Jewish doctors.

Herman Langbein, a political prisoner, wrote a landmark book about the people in Auschwitz including both the SS and the prisoners. He mentions Jewish doctors such as Perl, Nyiszli and Adelsberger. However, he does not go into any detail beyond anecdotes of functions or experiences. Weinberger provides an in-depth examination of inmate doctors of Auschwitz, particularly the Jewish doctors who worked in Block 10. Ley has not written exclusively on Jewish doctors in the extermination camps, concentrating instead on medicine in the era of National Socialism, sterilization and the medical profession and medicine in the concentration camps, particularly on medical crimes and neglect.[82] This secondary literature has provided the background to the medical system and the history of medicine and health in Auschwitz that has been invaluable to this work.

---

82 See A. Ley, Im Teufelskreis der Eugenik. Die Erfahrungen der Nürnbergerin Grete S. mit der NS- Erbpflege. In: *Bios* 12 (1999), pp. 92–107. M.M. Ruisinger (Ed.), *Gewissenlos – gewissenhaft. Menschenversuche im Konzentrationslager.* Ausstellungskatalog, Erlangen 2001. Nationalsozialistische Erbgesundheitspflege im Spannungsfeld gesellschaftlicher Interessen: Ideologische, ökonomische und medizinische Zielsetzungen bei der Zwangssterilisation. In S. Horn and P. Malina (Eds), *Medizin im Nationalsozialismus. Wege der Aufarbeitung*, Wien 2002, pp. 143–150. *Zwangssterilisation und Ärzteschaft. Hintergründe und Ziele ärztlichen Handelns 1934–1945*, New York, 2004. Medizin im Konzentrationslager: Gezielte Vernachlässigung, medizinische Minimalversorgung, ärztliche Verbrechen. Dauerausstellung in der Gedenkstätte Sachsenhausen. In: *Medizinhistorisches Journal*, 41, 2006.

Conclusion

I have not told you of our experiences to harrow you, but to strengthen you ... Now you may decide if you are justified in despairing.
Anonymous prisoner of Auschwitz (Des Pres 1976, 209)

After nine trips to Auschwitz over a number of years, I arrived for my final visit in December 2016. As was my custom, I arrived at 7:30 am. It was freezing cold and the staff were preparing for the expected stream of visitors. Walking on the cobblestones past the poplar trees and the blocks on either side I still could sense the presence of ghosts around me. Although the camp seemed the same, I had changed. The cloud of despair and sadness that hung over the camp whenever I had previously entered had partly lifted. Something had happened during my journey over those years that had altered my attitude towards death and survival. Within the available sources I had found out how the Jewish doctors survived Auschwitz. But in so doing, I had also discovered something about myself.

From the very beginning I knew I was facing years of research that would once again take me to the depths of inhumanity and evil that defied the imagination. I had already completed a book on Nazi medicine with a focus on human experiments. During that research I discovered Jewish doctors not only assisted the SS doctors in human experiments but they also worked in camp hospitals and infirmaries. This was particularly the case in Auschwitz, where my work was concentrated at the time. Initially I did not even contemplate pursuing the matter further but certain questions kept nagging at me. The most puzzling question, how the Jewish doctors survived an average of twenty months in hell, began as a curiosity but gradually became a passion.

Unfortunately, the work I commenced with such intense enthusiasm slowly became an untenable experience. I found I could not continue. The deeper I went into the subject, the more I relied on the memoirs and testimonials of survivors to find the answers. Everything I read and heard was to do with evil and its consequences, suffering, loss and death. Having read about the Nazi human experiments had brought to light the shocking cruelty and murder of children and reading these personal accounts of what happened in Auschwitz tore down any barriers that allowed me to learn of others' pain and horror without being subsumed in it. This of all of my work had a deep and lasting effect on me as a person, father and grandfather. I stopped writing because the emotional pain became too much to bear.

However, the nagging question of how the doctors survived would not leave me. It was a source of great frustration: I felt I had come so far and was so close to finding the answer to their survival yet I could not continue the work. That is

https://doi.org/10.1515/9783110598216-018

not until a chance meeting with a wise woman on a tram in Jerusalem. On my way back from giving a presentation on my survival model at Yad Vashem, I sat next to a woman who was attending the academic centre as a visiting scholar. She told me she had heard and was impressed by my presentation and theory. We discussed it for a while until I confessed that I had real doubts as to whether I would complete the work. She was curious so I explained my issues. Although she was sympathetic, she asked me two very frank questions: 'Have you known hard times before?' – to which I replied, 'Yes!'; and 'Did you get through those hard times?' – to which I replied, 'Yes!' She said, 'You will also get through this.'

Upon arriving home from Israel with this woman's voice in my head, I wondered how I was ever going to recommence writing. I began rearranging the memoirs of the survivors in my library and by chance I read a passage from Louis Micheels' memoir that became a defining moment for me: 'Very slowly I began to realize that I was actually free, my own master, once again a real person who did not need to fear that any moment might be the last' (Micheels 1989, 155).

I suddenly realized that I was not researching death. I was examining the quest for life! I started to reflect on some of the wonderful experiences I had had with the families of the survivors. When I was invited to the home of Sima Vaisman's nephew, Emanuel Marom, in Tel Aviv to interview him about his aunt, I found myself having dinner with twelve people, most of whom were relatives of Dr Vaisman. They spoke enthusiastically and lovingly about their aunt and of how she was the centre of the family, a person of wisdom and strength they could go to for support and comfort. Many memories rushed back to me about the joyous atmosphere of that night. We talked about a person who had lived, loved and was loved, and who had made a significant contribution to others' lives. She was the glue that held the family together.

The afternoon in Newton, Massachusetts, with the family of Louis Micheels, his wife Ina, son Ron and daughter Elizabeth and two of their children, Micheels' grandchildren, all spoke proudly of his life and career and how his lust for life continued well into his late eighties when he was still pursuing his favourite hobbies of woodwork, sailing and horse riding. The atmosphere of the home was so calm, quiet and friendly, much like the image I had of Louis.

My meetings with Ella and Giora, the daughter and grandson of Giselle Perl, were usually in a café in Haifa. Both spoke of the exciting times they spent with Giselle in New York and of their lives together in Israel once Giselle made Aliyah. They spoke of how proud they were of her not only for what she had achieved in surviving Auschwitz but of her accomplishments working in New York as an obstetrician and then volunteering in Shaare Zedek's gynaecology clinic in Jerusalem.

I thought of my meetings with Kalman in Tel Aviv. Sitting with this quiet gentle person telling me of his quest to find out why God did not protect the Jews and how he gained a Master's degree to help him get the answer from the Torah. He confessed he never got the answer but we had long discussions about the subject. He was full of life and proud of his accomplishments and his family.

And I went to the Sydney Jewish Museum and visited Lotte Weiz, a survivor of Auschwitz, who for two hours each Sunday is a guide. Lotte is now in her nineties, a vibrant, wonderful human being who is loved by everyone. She bears witness to thousands of visitors each year of life in Auschwitz and what evil humans can do. She has a purpose to her life.

I came to understand that to treat a subject such as the Holocaust and understand how one survives a death camp where almost everybody dies, it is first necessary to confront evil and its consequences, death and destruction. But it was also necessary to focus on the fact that some lived. This small group of Jewish doctors survived Auschwitz broken in body and spirit but they had beaten Hitler and his murderous intentions. I realized that if I was going to write about why and how these people survived they would want me to tell the story not only of the conditions, suffering and cruelty but also of how they attempted to save lives, and how they were driven to live so as to bear witness and ensure that in the future such inhumanity would never be repeated. The very fact that so many Jewish doctors who survived Auschwitz wrote memoirs of their life and work in Auschwitz is proof of their compulsion to bear witness. The tragedy is that, despite their efforts as witnesses of what the Nazis attempted and the lesson of what evil lurks in ordinary people, we have not learned from history. We have just given it a name: Genocide.

The main legacy from this study is the conception of a model of how to survive extreme adversity over a long period of time. However, what is of greater significance is the treasure trove of information about the human condition, which the study of the survival of this small group of people has provided. What we have learnt is that the essentials of life are necessary for survival and that each of us has personal traits that determine our strengths and weaknesses and govern our ability to cope with adversity. The surviving doctors showed personal traits that rendered them seemingly indestructible. We have found that there is a relationship between early childhood and adolescence and such personal traits as resilience, hardiness and self-esteem, and learnt that a childhood where family love, support and security are provided is more likely to foster these traits. We have discovered that communication and forming and maintaining relationships are essential to emotional health, to protecting one's identity and maintaining humanity. We have observed the crucial importance of defence mechanisms that allow the victim to become preoccupied and to derive some respite or protection from the daily trauma. These are lessons we can learn from the life and work of the Jewish doctors who survived the camps.

Tragically the survivor often becomes a captive of the traumatic events of the past. Delbo reminds the reader that those who survived Auschwitz do not leave it unmarked and that to continue to survive, they must adjust:

> I have returned
> from a world beyond knowledge
> and now must unlearn,
> for otherwise I clearly see
> I can no longer live. Delbo (1995, xv)

Micheels' wife told me that during the early years of their married life Louis had terrible nightmares. While he refused to speak of them, she knew they were from his days in Auschwitz. Vaisman maintained her rage against the Germans until very late in her life and spoke very little of her experiences in the camp. For many, life after Auschwitz continued to be a struggle. Who could witness and be subject to such inhumanity without irreparable damage? Some survivors such as Primo Levi and Jean Améry committed suicide. The specific reason why they took their lives is unknown but it may be as a result of their inability to cope with the nightmares, memories and despair they carried with them like heavy chains. It may have been because in reality very little if anything had changed. If they were alive today and reflected on the past atrocities such as Rwanda, Bosnia, Cambodia and Darfur and the recent attempted genocide in Sudan, Rohingya, the Yazidis, and the Shia Muslims amongst other minorities, after surviving Auschwitz they would lose all hope that history won't be repeated. We are now in the first quarter of the 21st century and anti-semitism is rising, the Middle East is in chaos and millions are homeless and dying from starvation, epidemics and being slaughtered and the number of refugees is countless. Right-wing governments have been elected throughout Europe and now in the Americas including North America led by charismatic leaders bringing with them anti-racial, anti-religious and right wing ideological policies.

The Holocaust was an evil visited upon the Jewish people. It has become symbolic of everything destructive, murderous and catastrophic. Before I commenced this project, I was asked to describe what the Holocaust meant to me and I replied, 'Death, loss, suffering, children, flames' and so on. Because I had visited Auschwitz and many memorial museums I could and can see piles of shoes, suitcases, reading glasses and so many other awful images. While these images are with me still, I now have positive thoughts as well. I have hope. I think the account of the survival of the doctors is one of inspiration and testimony to the extraordinary courage, resilience and goodness of ordinary people. I now know that, given the right circumstances, the possession of strong personal traits and the determination to protect one's self against the maelstrom of fear and evil, it is possible to survive adversity.

My journey, as difficult as it has been, has provided me the opportunity to understand more about the human condition and that irrespective of what we are we are driven by who we are particularly under conditions of extreme adversity. That as ordinary humans we are fragile, vulnerable, weak, dishonest, manipulative and capable of cruelty and murder particularly when our life or our loved one's life is at risk. The decisions and actions by the Jewish doctors in Auschwitz and to take it further all Jewish prisoners in the camps and ghettoes were human. The label they were given, doctors, lawyers, accountants and so on before Hitler came to power did not apply during his murderous reign and particularly in the camps. The Jewish doctor's life in the camps, such as Auschwitz, was a complete paradox. On the one hand the doctor strove to uphold the tenet to protect the patient yet on the other hand they were driven by the innate compulsion to survive. In many cases the decisions to survive led to suffering and sometimes the death of patients they were committed to protect. Under the circumstances none of the actions or decisions by the doctors can be judged.

I have only known these doctors for a short five years but I feel I have known them all my life. They have become my companions and they live with me every day inspiring me with their courage and their ability to overcome overwhelming odds. Although I know they were in a very dark place, when I think of them and their life after Auschwitz they were still never free and were troubled and traumatised but they were with their families and friends new and old. They survived and slowly rebuilt their lives. I imagine Louis in a smart suit lecturing to a classroom of eager medical students at Yale not standing in thin pyjamas deciding who was to be selected for phenol injections. I see Giselle beaming as she proudly assists another baby into the world at the neonatal clinic in Jerusalem not performing an abortion on the filthy floor of an overcrowded hut. I picture Sima in a Parisian café chatting away with her friends, nieces and nephews after a long day in her surgery not an emaciated thirty-kilo waif comforting a prisoner about to take their last breath. The doctors do not talk of that other place. But they remembered.

I look upon them all as extraordinary people but I know they were ordinary folk who were forced into unimaginable circumstances and survived. These special friends of mine are with me as a constant source of inspiration and a reminder that it is possible to beat insurmountable odds and survive.

Epilogue

When I was 17 years old, I spent my mid-year university break working on an assembly line with a man who was in his late 30s. Over the past fifty years I have often wondered what became of him. He was unkempt, unshaven, and sometimes arrived at work not drunk but smelling of alcohol. He didn't seem to eat at morning tea or lunch breaks, settling instead for a cigarette. He never acknowledged or spoke to me and never mixed with any of the other workers. He did, however, protect me on the line that involved powerful cutting machinery. He watched over me like a mother hen. He didn't speak, he just watched and acted when I got too close to the blades. I felt safe. Out of interest I asked one of the workers who had been at the factory for some time if he knew anything about the guy, about what was wrong with him. He told me he had been a young doctor when his wife and young child had been killed in a motor accident. He never recovered. The owner of the business knew the family and gave him a job. He had become an alcoholic.

I was overcome with sadness and couldn't understand why after so much time he wasn't able to try and rebuild his life. Like the Muselmänner, he was obviously alive but not living. What happened to him? I now know about life and the experience of adversity, loss and tragedy. Life is not that simple. The question I now ask myself is how I would react at the tragic loss of my wife and child in such circumstances.

Nothing can compare to the experiences of those who suffered at the hands of the Nazis in the ghettos and camps during the Holocaust. However, adversity, loss and tragedy are universal. We all face one or more such challenges at some time in our lives. How we meet them is of the greatest importance.

Let us look at my co-worker. He was in his own hell experiencing every person's fear. Yet he had someone who cared for him – his boss and friend, and had the essentials of life to stay alive. He had work, even if it was not his profession. Perhaps the repetitive boring nature of his work gave him too much time to think and added to his despair rather than giving him respite and protection from his demons. Did he have the will to live? Was he willing to call for help from family and friends and professional help? Did he have the determination and resilience to suffer and overcome further pain? Or did he make the choice to shut himself off and stop living?

Adversity is relative but has the same effect. It is similar to gas in a bottle. Small amounts of gas fill the bottle the same as large amounts. They both completely fill the bottle. The same applies to grief and loss. The difference is how adversity is managed and survival takes place.

https://doi.org/10.1515/9783110598216-019

Just as the Jewish doctors consciously or unconsciously followed a construct to endure adversity and survive indescribable inhumanity, ordinary people in this complex world need the tools to survive tragedy and adversity if and when it arrives – not only to stay alive but also to try and live a productive and full life.

My co-worker who I never got to know was prevented from 'living' because he appeared not to have the will to live; of the three pillars for survival one or two were missing.

Bibliography

Adelsberger, L 1969, *Auschwitz: A Doctor's Story*, Robson Books, London.

Affleck, G, & Tennen, H 1996, Construing benefits from adversity: Adaptational significance and dispositional underpinnings. Journal of Personality, 64, 899–922

Albright, M 2012, *Prague Winter: A Personal Story of Remembrance and War 1937–1948*, Harper Collins, New York.

Allen, JG 2005, *Coping with Trauma: Hope through Understanding*, American Psychiatric Publishing, Washington, DC.

Alvarez, J & Hunt, M 2005. Risk and resilience in canine search and rescue handlers after 9/11. Journal of Traumatic Stress, 18, 497–505

Améry, J 1986, *At the Mind's Limit: Contemplations by a Survivor on Auschwitz and Its Realities*, Schecken Books, New York.

Anderson, T 1993, *Den of Lions: Memoirs of Seven Years*, Crown Publishers Inc, New York.

Anderson, N. B & Anderson. P. E 2003. Emotional longevity: what really determines how long you live? Viking: New York

Arad, Y, Gutman, Y & Margaliot, A (eds) 1990, *Documents on the Holocaust: Selected Sources on the Destruction of the Jews of Germany and Austria, Poland and the Soviet Union*, Yad Vashem, Jerusalem.

Arad, Y (ed) 1990, *The Pictorial History of the Holocaust*, Macmillan, New York.

American Psychiatric Association (APA) 2000, *Diagnostic & Statistical Manual of Mental Disorders* (revised 4th ed.), APA, Washington, DC.

Arendt, H 1948, 'The concentration camps', *Partisan Review*, July 15, pp. 743.

Auluc A, Pai, KM 2005, 'Noma: life cycle of a devastating sore – case report and literature review, *Journal of the Canadian Dental Association*, vol. 71, no.10, pp. 757.

Auschwitz-Birkenau State Museum Archives 1947, transcripts of the trial of Rudolf Höss, Vol.22, Auschwitz-Birkenau State Museum, Oświećim.

Auschwitz-Birkenau State Museum Archives 1946, *Medical Science Abused: German Medical Science as Practiced in Concentration Camps and in the so-called Protectorate*, reported by Czechoslovak doctors, Auschwitz-Birkenau State Museum, Oświećim.

Auschwitz: Inside the Nazi State 2005, documentary, BBC. Directed by Laurence Rees & Catherine Tatge.

Bankhalter, S 1992, Oral history interview of Sam Bankhalter, USHMM, Accession no. 1994.A.0447.5, RG no., RG-50.042.0005.

Bankier, D & Gutman, I (eds) 2003, *Nazi Europe and the Final Solution*, The Holocaust Martyrs' and Heroes' Remembrance Authority, Yad Vashem, Jerusalem.

Bankier, D & Michman, D (eds) 2008, *Holocaust: Historiography in Context*, Emergence, *Challenges*, Polemics & Achievements, Yad Vashem, Jerusalem.

Barkai, A 1989, *From Boycott to Annihilation*, University Press of New England, London.

Bar On, K 2010, interview with Ross Halpin, 30 March, Tel Aviv.

Bartov, O (ed) 2000, *Holocaust: Origins, Implementations, Aftermath*, Routledge, London.

Bauer, Y 1982, *A History of the Holocaust*, Franklin Watts, New York.

Bauer, Y 2002, *Rethinking the Holocaust*, Yale University Press, New Haven, CT.

Baumslag, N 1995, *Murderous Medicine*, Praeger Publishers, West Port, CT.

Beauchamp, TL & Walters, L 2003, *Contemporary Issues in Bioethics*, 6th ed, Thomson Wadsworth, Belmont, CA.

https://doi.org/10.1515/9783110598216-020

Beaton. R Murphy. S Johnson. C Pike. K & Corneil. W 1999 Coping responses and postraumatic stress symptomatology in urban fire service personnel. Journal of Traumatic Stress, 12, 293–308

Beijlin, A 1961, Written memoirs of Dr Aaron Beijlin, document 1741/147 – 032039, Yad Vashem Archives, Jerusalem.

Benedict, S & Georges, J 2006, 'Nurses and the sterilization experiments of Auschwitz: a postmodernist perspective', *Advances in Nursing Scien*ce, vol. 1, no.4, pp. 277.

Benedict, S & Georges, J 2006, 'An ethics of testimony: prisoner nurses at Auschwitz', *Advances in Nursing Science*, vol. 29, no. 2, pp.161.

Berger, N (ed.) 1995, *Jews and Medicine: Religion, Culture*, Science, Jewish Publication Society, Jerusalem.

Bettelheim, B 1960, *The Informed Heart: Autonomy in a Mass Age*, Free Press of Glencoe, New York.

Bezwińska, J 1972, *KL Auschwitz Seen by the SS: Höss, Broad, Kremer*, Państwowe Muzeum, Oświęcim.

Birenbaum, H 2009, *Hope is the Last to Die:* State Museum Oświęcim.

Bloch, GR 1999, *The Holocaust*. Red Hen Press, Los Angeles, CA.

Bloch, H 1947, 'The Personality of Inmates of Concentration Camps', *American Journal of Sociology*, vol. 1.

Bluhm, H 1999, 'How did they survive? Mechanisms of defence in Nazi concentration camps', *American Journal of Psychotherapy*, vol. 53, no. 1.

Blum, H (ed) 1985, *Defence and Resistance*, International Universities Press, New York.

Borowski, T 1976, *This Way for the Gas, Ladies and Gentlemen*, Penguin, New York.

Boss, P 2006, *Loss Trauma and Resilience: Therapeutic Work with Ambiguous Loss*, WW Norton & Co, New York.

Braham R 1994, *The Politics of Genocide: The Holocaust in Hungary*, vol. 2, Columbia University Press, New York.

Breitman, R 1991, *The Architect of Genocide: Himmler and the Final Solution*, Bodley Head, London.

Broszat, M 1965, 'Nationalsozialistische Konzentrationslager 1933–1945′, in Buchheim et al. (eds) *Anatomie des SS-Staates*, vol.2, Walter Verlag, Olten.

Browning, CR 1998, *Ordinary Men: Reserve Police Battalion 101 and the Final Solution in Poland*, Harper Collins, New York.

Browning, CR 2000, *Nazi Policy, Jewish Workers, German Killers*, University Press, Cambridge.

Browning, CR 2010, *Remembering Survival: Inside a Nazi-Labor Camp*, WW Norton & Co, New York.

Browning, CR 2000, *The Origins of the Final Solution: The Evolution of Nazi Jewish Policy, September 1939 - March 1942*, Yad Vashem, Jerusalem.

Browning, CR 1992, *The Path to Genocide: Essays on Launching the Final Solution*, University Press, Cambridge.

Brozan N 1982, 'Out of Death, A Zest for life,' *New York Times*, 15 November.

Camus, A 2009, *The Plague*, Penguin Books, Camberwell, Victoria.

Caplan, AL (ed) 1992, *When Medicine Went Mad*, Humana Press, Totowa, New Jersey.

Carver. C S Pozo. C Harris. S. D Noriega. V Scheier. M F Robinson. D. S et al. 1993 How coping mediates the effect of optimism on distress: A study of women with early stage of breast cancer. Journal of Personality and Social Psychology, 65 375–390

Clend innen, I 1998, *Reading the Holocaust*, Text Publishing Company, Melbourne.

Chess, S & Hertzig, M (eds) 1990, *Annual Progress in Child* Psychiatry *and* Child Development, Brunner Mazel, Philadelphia.

Chimino, L 1984, Written testimony of Lucy Chimino, document 0-3/5114, Yad Vashem Archives, Jerusalem.

Cogon, E 2006, *The Theory and Practice of Hell: The German Concentration Camps and the Systems behind Them*, Farrar, Straus & Giroux, New York.

Cohen, EA 1973, *The Abyss: A Confession*, WW Norton & Co, New York.

Cowley, C 2008, *Medical Ethics, Ordinary Concepts and Ordinary Lives*, Palgrave, New York.

Cramer, P 2009, 'Seven Pillars of Defence Mechanism Theory', *Proceedings of the Annual Meeting of the Rapaport-Klein Study Group*, Austen Riggs Center, Stockbridge, Massachusetts, viewed 6 January 2010, www.psychology.sunysb.edu/attachment/rapaportklein/bobholt/bobholtphotos.pdf

Cramer, P 1996, *The Development of Defence Mechanisms: Theory, Research and* Assessment, Springer Verlag, New York.

Cyran, HB 1984, *Inside Auschwitz: Written in Blood, a Personal Memory*, Child & Henry Publishing, Brookvale, NSW.

Czech, D 1990, *Auschwitz Chronicle 1939–1945: From the Archives of the Auschwitz Memorial and the German Federal Archives*, Oxford University Press, New York.

Dante, A 1995, *The Divine Comedy* New York: Random House Aligieri 2010, *Inferno*, Penguin, London.

Dawidowicz, L 1975, *The War Against the Jews, 1933–45*, Penguin, New York.

Dawidowicz, L 1981, *The Holocaust and the Historians*, Harvard University Press, Cambridge, MA.

D'Antonio, P 2006, *Nursing History Review*, Springer Publishing Company, New York.

De Beauvoir, S 1948, *Ethics of Ambiguity*, Citadel Press, Secaucus, NJ.

Delbo, C 1986, *None of Us Will Return*, Grove Publishing, New York.

Delbo, C 1995, *Auschwitz and After*, Yale University Press, London.

Des Pres, T 1976, *The Survivor: An Anatomy of Life in the Death Camps*, Oxford University Press, New York.

Didi-Huberman, G 2008, *Images In Spite of All: Four Photographs from Auschwitz*, University of Chicago, IL.

Donat, A 1958, *The Holocaust Kingdom*, Farrar, Straus & Giroux, New York.

Doob, LW 1978, *Panorama of Evil: Insights from Behavioural Sciences*, Greenwood Press, Westport, CT.

Drix, S 1995, *Witness: A Holocaust Memoir*, Fountain Paperbacks, London.

Dvorjetski, M 1952, 'The Jewish medical resistance and Nazi criminal medicine during the disastrous period'. *Lecture at the World Jewish Medical Congress in Jerusalem*, transcript held at Yad Vashem Library, Jerusalem.

Dwork, D 1995, 'Lamed-Vovniks of Twentieth-Century Europe: Participants in Jewish child rescue', in Geyer, M & Boyer, JW (eds), *Resistence against Third Reich 1933–1990*, University of Chicago Press Chicago.

Edelman, M 2016, *The Ghetto Fights: Warsaw 1943–45*, Bookmarks Publishing, London.

Efron, JM 2001, *Medicine and the German Jews: A History*, Yale University Press, New Haven, CT.

Efron, JM 1994, *Defenders of the Race: Jewish Doctors & Race Science in Fin-De-Siècle Europe*, Yale University Press, New Haven, CT.

Eisenberg, N, Valiente, C & and Champion, C 2004, 'Empathy-Related Responding: Moral, Social and Socialization Correlates', in Miller, AG (ed), *The Social Psychology of Good and Evil*, Guilford Press, New York.

Ehrenreich, E 2007, 'Otmar von Verschuer and the "scientific" legitimization of Nazi anti-Jewish policy', *Holocaust and Genocide Studies*, vol. 21, no.1.

Elias, R 1998, *Triumph of Hope: From Theresienstadt and Auschwitz to Israel*, John Wiley & Sons, New York.

Falstein, L (ed) 1963, *The Martyrdom of Jewish Doctors in Poland*, Exposition Press Inc, New York.

Fejkiel, W 1971, *Auschwitz Anthology*, vol. 2, part 1, *Health Service in the Auschwitz I Concentration Camp*, 4–37, International Auschwitz Committee, Warsaw.

Fejkiel, W 1994, *Więźniarski Szpital W KL Auschwitz*, Wydawnictwo Państwowego Muzeum, Oświęcim.

Figes, O 2012, *Just Send Me Word: A True Story of Love and Survival in the Gulag*, Allen Lane, London.

Fine, S 1991, 'Resilience and human adaptability: Who rises above adversity?', *American Journal of Occupational Therapy*, 45, pp. 493.

Fischer, K 1998, *The History of an Obsession: German Judeophobia and the Holocaust*, Continuum Publishing Company, New York.

Fleck, L 1958, Testimony of Professor Dr Ludwik Fleck, bacteriologist, document 0-3/650, Yad Vashem Archives, Jerusalem.

Folkman. S & Moskowitz J. T 2000. Positive affect and the other side of coping. American Psychologist, 55, 647–654

Frankl, V 1959, *From Death Camp to Existentialism*, Beacon Press, Boston.

Frankl, V 1959, *Man's Search for Meaning*, Washington Square Press, New York.

Freidenreich, HP 1996, 'Jewish women physicians in central Europe in the early twentieth century', *Contemporary Jewry*, vol. 17, no. 1.

Freud, A 1966, *The Ego and the Mechanisms of Defence*, Hogarth Press, London.

Friedländer, S 1984, 'From antisemitism to extermination: a historiographical study of Nazi policies toward the Jews and an essay in interpretation', *Yad Vashem Studies*, vol. 16.

Friedländer, S 1997, *Nazi Germany and the Jews: The Years of Persecution 1933–1939*, Harper Collins, New York.

Friedländer, S 1997, *Nazi Germany and the Jews 1939–1945: The Years of Extermination*, Harper Collins, New York.

Friedländer, S 1993, *Memory, History and the Extermination of the Jews of Europe*, Indiana University Press, Indianapolis, IN.

Friedman, AJ (ed) 1980, *Roads to Extinction: Essays on the Holocaust*, Jewish Publication Society of America, New York.

Fritsch, T 1919, *Handbuch der Judenfrage*, Sleipner, Hamburg.

Garmezy, N 1985, 'Stress-resistant children: The search for protective factors', in Stevenson, JE (ed), *Recent Research In Developmental Psychopathology*, Pergamon, NY.

Garliński, J 1975, *Fighting Auschwitz: The Resistance Movement in the Concentration Camp*, Fawcett Crest Books, Greenwich, CT.

Garrard, E & Scarre, G (eds) 2003, *Moral Philosophy and the Holocaust*, Ashgate Publishing Company, Aldershot, England.

Geyer, M & Boyer, JW (eds) 1995, *Resistance against the Third Reich 1933–1990*, Chicago University Press, Chicago, IL.

Gilbert, M 1987, *The Holocaust: The Jewish Tragedy*, Fontana Press, London.

Glover, G 1977, *Causing Death and Saving Lives*, Penguin Books, New York.

Goldenberg, E 1995, oral testimony, accessed at University of Southern California Shoah Foundation, Oral History/VHA Interview Code: 3478.

Goldenberg, J n.d. 'Explanations for Survival by Jewish Survivors of the Holocaust' viewed 24 June 2018, https://www.scribd.com/document/219502505/Explanations-for-Survival-by-Jewish-Survivors-of-the-Holocaust-Goldenberg

Goldie, P & Copland, A (eds) 2012, *Empathy: Philosophical and Psychological Perspectives*, Oxford University Press, Oxford.

Götz, A, Chroust, P & Pross, C 1994, *Cleansing the Fatherland: Nazi Medicine and Racial Hygiene*, John Hopkins University Press, London.

Grief, G 2005, *We Wept Without Tears: Testimonies of the Jewish Sonderkommandos from Auschwitz*, Yale University Press, New Haven, CT.

Grodin, MA 2010, 'Mad, Bad, or Evil: How Doctors Turn to Torture and Murder', in Rubenfeld, S (ed), *Medicine after the Holocaust: From the Master Race to the Human Genome and Beyond*, Palgrave, New York.

Grünberg, P 2007, 'Zur Geschichte des Lagers Auschwitz-Monowitz (BUNA)', interview with Curt Posner, 16 June, *Interviews with Buna/Monowitz Concentration Camp Survivors*, viewed 23 June 2018, http://www.wollheim-memorial.de/en/paul_gruenberg

Gruner, W 2006, *Jewish Forced Labor under the Nazis: Economic Needs and Racial Aims, 1938–1944*, Cambridge University Press, New York.

Gutman, Y & Berenbaum, M 1998, *Anatomy of the Auschwitz Death Camps*, Indiana University Press, Bloomington, IN.

Haas, A 1984, *The Doctor and the Damned*, St Martin's Press, New York.

Haffner, D 1946, *Aspects Pathologiques du Camp de Concentration D'Auschwitz – Birkenau*, Imprimerie Union Co-Operative, Tours.

Haglund. M, E Nestadt. P, S Cooper. N, S Southwick. S. M & Charney. D, S 2007. Psychobiological mechanism of resilience: Relevance to prevention and treatment of stress-related Psychopathology. Development and Psychopathology, 19, 889–920

Halpin, RW 2011, *A Matter of Concern: The Ethical Dilemma of Using Nazi Medical Research Data*, Südwestdeutscher Verlag, Saarbrücken.

Hart, K 1981, *Return to Auschwitz: The Remarkable Life of a Girl Who Survived the Holocaust*, Sidgwick & Jackson, London.

Hartman H 1958, *Ego Psychology and the Problem of Adaptation*, International Universities Press, New York.

Herbert, U (ed) 2000, *National Socialist Extermination Policies: Contemporary German Perspectives and Controversies*, Berghahn Books, New York.

Hilberg, R 1996, *The Politics of Memory: The Journey of a Holocaust Historian*, Ivan R Dee, Chicago.

Hilberg, R 1985, *The Destruction of the European Jews*, vols. 1, 2 & 3, Holmes & Meier, New York.

Hill, M & Williams, LN 1966, *Auschwitz in England*, Panther Books, London.

Hobsbawn, EJ 1087, *The Age of Empire, 1875–1914*, Pantheon Books, London.

Hoge. E, A Austin. E, D & Pollock M. H 2007. Resilience: Research evidence and conceptual consideration for post traumatic stress disorder, Depression and Anxiety, 24, 139–152

Holocaust Education and Archive Research Team, 2013 'The Auschwitz-Birkenau and Sub-Camps. Evacuation and the Death Marches – January 1945', viewed 1 March 2012, https//www.holocaustresearchproject.org/othercamps/auschdeathmarch.html/

Höss, R 1996, *Death Dealer: Memoirs of the SS Kommandant at Auschwitz*, Da Capo Press, New York.

International Auschwitz Committee [IAC], 2002 *Auschwitz: Anthology*, vols. 1 & 2, IAC, Warsaw.

International Auschwitz Committee [IAC] 1986, *Nazi Medicine: Doctors, Victims and Medicine in Auschwitz*, Howard Fertig, New York.

International Tracing Service (ITS) 2011 Archives, Details outlining movement of Dr Vaisman from Auschwitz to Ravensbrück, January 1945, to Neustadt-Glewe, a German town, in Mecklenburg-Western Pomerania, in the district of Ludwigslust in February 1945, Correspondence Form 181, accessed at the ITS, Bad Arolsen, Germany.

International Tracing Service (ITS) 2011 Archives, Transport list, doc. 86826612 no.1, 6. 3.32/120001.../142801.../0142984/3Korresponenz-Akte T/D – 142984, accessed at the ITS, Bad Arolsen, Germany.

Jacobs, B 1959, *The Dentist of Auschwitz: a Memoir*, Kentucky University Press, Lexington, Kentucky.

Jacobs, JL (ed) 2009, *The Holocaust: Voices of Scholars*, Centre for Holocaust Studies, Jagiellonian University, Kraków.

Johnsen. B. H Eid. J Laberg. J. C & Thayer. J. E 2002 The effect of sensitizization and oping style on post-traumatic stress symptoms and quality of life: Two longitudinal studies. Scandinavian Journal of Psychology, 43, 181–188

Kahana, E, Kahana, B, Harel, Z & Rosner, T 1988, 'Coping with extreme trauma', in Wilson, J et al (eds), *Human Adaptation to Extreme Stress: from the Holocaust to Vietnam*, Plenum Press, New York.

Kater, MH 1989, *Doctors Under Hitler*, University of North Carolina Press, Chapel Hill, CA.

Kazerne Dossin n.d., *History – the Transports*, Kazerne Dossin, Mechelen, Belgium, viewed 31 July 2011, www.cicbe.be/en/content/transports

Kent, M & Davis, M 2010, 'The Emergence of Capacity-Building Programs and Models of Resilience, Zautra, A & Hall, JS (eds), *Handbook of Adult Resilience*, Guilford Press, New York.

Kernberg, O 1991, 'The psychopathology of hatred', *Journal of the American Psychoanalytic Association*, vol. 39, pp. 99.

Kershaw, I 2008, *Hitler, the Germans and the Final Solution*, Yale University Press, New Haven, CT.

Kielar, W 1981, *Anus Mundi: Five Years in Auschwitz, a Personal Record*, Allen Lane, London.

Kielar, W n.d., from memoirs of Wieslaw Kielar, prisoner number 290, Auschwitz-Birkenau State Museum Recollections Fond, vol. 64., pp. 221, Auschwitz-Birkenau State Museum, Oswiecim.

Koenig. H. G George. L, K & Titus. P 2004 Religious, spirituality, and health in medically ill hospitalized older patients. Journal of the American Geriatric Society, 52, 554–562

Koonz, C 2003, *The Nazi Conscience*, Harvard University Press, Cambridge, MA.

KKoenig, H & Kohák, E 1973, *The Victors and the Vanquished*, Horizon Press, New York.

Kozub, B 2009, 'A discussion of the conservation of "SS-Hygiene Institute" documents in the archives of the Auschwitz-Birkenau State Museum' in Proceedings of the Book and Paper Group session, AIC 37th Annual Meeting, 20–23 May, Los Angeles, CA, viewed 23 June 2018, https://cool.conservation-us.org/coolaic/sg/bpg/annual/v28/bp28-08.pdf

Kraus, E & Yardeni, G 2011, Interviews with Ross Halpin on 4 April and 5 November, Haifa, Israel.

Kraus, O & Kulka, E 1966, *The Death Mills of Auschwitz*, Jerusalem Post printing, Jerusalem.

Kubica, H 2006, *The Extermination at KL Auschwitz of Poles Evicted from the Zamość Region in the Years 1942–1943*, Auschwitz- Birkenau State Museum, Oświęcim.

Kwiet, K Designing Survival: A Graphic Artist in Birkenau in Matth

Lagnado, LM & Cohn Dekel S 1991, *Children of the Flames: Dr Josef Mengele and the Untold Story of the Twins of Auschwitz*, Penguin, New York.

Landau, RS 1998, *Studying the Holocaust: Issues, Readings and Documents*, Routledge, London.

Langbein, H 2004, *People in Auschwitz*, University of North Carolina, Chapel Hill, NC.

Langbein, H 1994 *Against All Hope: Resistance in the Nazi Concentration* Camps *1938 – 1945*, Paragon House, New York.

Langer, LL 1991, *Holocaust Testimonies: The Ruins of Memory*,Yale University Press, New Haven, CT.

Langer, LL 1982, *Versions of Survival: The Holocaust and the Human Spirit*, State University of the New York Press, Albany.

Lasik, A, Piper, F, Setkiewicz, P & Strzelecka, I 2000, *Auschwitz 1940–1945: Central Issues in the History of the Camp*, volume 1, Auschwitz State Museum, Oświęcim.

Lawrence, DH 2008, Birds, Beasts & Flowers Poems, David R. Godine, Jaffrey, New Hampshire

Lazarus, R & Folkman S 1984, *Stress, Appraisal and Coping*, Springer, New York.

Le Bon, G 1968, *The Crowd: A Study of the Popular Mind*, NS Berg, Dunwoody, GA.

Lengyel, O 1995, *Five Chimneys: A Woman Survivor's True Story of Auschwitz*, Academy Chicago Publishers, Chicago, IL.

Levi, P 1989, *The Drowned and the Saved*, Abacus, London.

Levi, P 1995, *The Reawakening*, Simon & Schuster, New York.

Levi, P 1996, *Survival in Auschwitz: The Nazi Assault on Humanity* Touchstone, New York.

Lichtenberg, J & Slap J 1972, 'On the defence mechanism: A survey and synthesis', *Journal of the American Psychoanalytic Association*, vol. 20.

Lifton, J R 2000, *The Nazi Doctors: Medical Killing and the Psychology of Genocide*, Basic Books, Washington.

Lipstadt, L 2011, *The Eichmann Trial*, Schocken Books, New York.

Loewald, H 1988, *Sublimation: Inquiries into Theoretical Psychoanalysis*, Yale University Press, New Haven, CT.

Lohalm U 2000, 'Local Administration and Nazi Anti-Jewish Policy', in Bankier, D (ed), *Probing the Depth of German Antisemitism*, Yad Vashem, Jerusalem.

Longerich, P 2010, *Holocaust: The Nazi Persecution and Murder of the Jews*, Oxford University Press, Oxford.

Longerich, P 2003, *The Unwritten Order: Hitler's Role in the Final Solution*, Tempus Publishing Limited, Gloucestershire.

Lord Russell of Liverpool 1962, *The Trial of Adolf Eichmann*, William Heinemann, London.

Lorska, D 1971, 'Block D in Auschwitz', in International Auschwitz Committee [IAC], *Auschwitz: Anthology*, vol. 1, Part 2, IAC, Warsaw.

Lowy, A 2011, interview with Ross Halpin on 11 April, Sydney.

Madajczyk, C 1970, *Polityka III Rzeszy w okupowanej Polsce*, vol. 2, Panstwowy Instytut Warschau, Warsaw.

Madajczyk, C (ed) 1977, *Inter Arma Non Silent Musae: The War and Culture, 1939–1945*, Panstwowy Instytut Warschau, Warsaw.

Manne. S Duhamel. K Ostrofr. J Parsons. S Martini. R Williams. S, F et al. 2003 Coping and a mother's depressive symptoms during and after pediatric bone marrow transplantation. Journal of the American Academy of Child Adolescent Psychiatry, 42, 1055–1068

Manvell, R & Frankel, H 2007, *Heinrich Himmler: the SS, Gestapo, His Life and Career*, WW Norton & Co, New York.

Matthäus, J (ed) 2009, *Approaching an Auschwitz Survivor: Holocaust Testimony and Its Transformation*, Oxford University Press, Oxford.

Marmar, ER & Horowitz, M J 1988, 'Post Traumatic Stress Disorder' in Wilson, JP Harel, Z & Kahana, D (eds), *Human Adaption to Extreme Stress: from the Holocaust to Vietnam*, Plenum, New York.

Marom, E 2011, interview with Ross Halpin, 12 January, Tel Aviv.

May, E 1943, Report to the Ahnenerbeinstitut, NS 21/7999, Heft 202 – APMAB.12 – Koblencja Vol.2 pp. 173–175, Bundisarchiv Koblenz, Germany.

May, L & Kohn, J (eds) 2006, *Hannah Arendt: Twenty Years Later*, MIT Press, Cambridge, MA.

Mayer, J & Faber, M 2010, 'Personal Intelligence and Resilience: Recovery in the Shadow of Broken Connections', in Reich, J, Zautra, A & Hall, JS (eds), *Handbook of Adult Resilience*, Guilford Press, New York.

Mazower, M 2009, *Hitler's Empire: Nazi Rule in Occupied Europe*, Penguin, London.

McCain, J 2008, 'Prisoner of War: A First-Person Account,' *US News & World Report*, January 28.

McCullough, ML Hoyt, WT Larson, DB& Koenig, HG 2000. Religious involvement and mortality: A meta-analytic review. Health Psychology,19, 211–222.

McFarland-Icke, BR 1999, *Nurses in Nazi Germany: Moral Choice in History*, Princeton University Meissner, W. W. (1970). Notes on identification: f i Origins in Freud. The Psychoanalytic Quarterly, 39, 563-589, Princeton, NJ.

Meichenbaum, D 1985 Stress Inoculation training. New York: Pergamon Press

Mencius 1963, *The Book of Mencius: from a Source Book in Chinese Philosophy*, translated by Wing-Tsit Chan, Princeton University Press, Princeton, NJ.

Michael, R & Doerr, K 2002, *Nazi-Deutsch – Nazi German: An English Lexicon of the Language of the Third Reich*, Greenwood Press, Westport, CT.

Michalczyk, JJ (ed) 1994, *Medicine Ethics and the Third Reich: Historical and Contemporary Issues*, Sheed & Ward, Kansas City, MO.

Micheels, LJ 1989, *Doctor 117647: a Holocaust Memoir: a Psychoanalyst's Moving Account of His Experiences in the Nazi Death Camps*, Yale University Press, New Haven, CT.

Milgram, S 1974, *Obedience to Authority: an Experimental View*, Harper & Row, New York.

Miller, A (ed) 1996, *The Bell Shakespeare*, Science Press, Marrickville, NSW.

Miller, A 2004, *The Social Psychology of Good and Evil*, Guilford Press, New York.

Minney, R 1966, *I Shall Fear No Evil: the Story of Dr Alina Brewda's Survival in Auschwitz*, Corgi Books, London.

Mitscherlich, A & Mielke, F 1949 *Doctors of Infamy: the Story of the Nazi Medical Crimes*, Henry Schuman, New York.

Mitscherlich, A & Mielke, F 1949, *Medizin ohne Menschlichkeit, Dokumente des Nürnberger Ärzteprozesses*, Fischer Taschenbuchverlag, Frankfurt.

Monroe, K 2004, *The Hand of Compassion: Portraits of Moral Choice during the Holocaust*, Princeton University Press, Princeton, NJ.

Mostowicz, A 2005, *With a Yellow Star and a Red Cross: aDoctor in the Lódź Ghetto*, Valentine Mitchell, Middlesex.

Müller-Hill, B 1998, *Murderous Science: Elimination by Scientific Selection of Jews, Gypsies and Others in Germany, 1933–1945*, Cold Spring Laboratory Press, New York.

Musial, B 2000, 'The origins of "Operation Reinhard": the decision-making process for the mass murder of the Jews in the Generalgouvernement', *Yad Vashem Studies*, vol. 28.

Musiot, J 2001, *Man and Crime*, Auschwitz-Birkenau Museum, Oświęcim.

Nadav, DS 2009, *Medicine and Nazism*, Hebrew University Press, Jerusalem.

Newman, JS 1964, *In the Hell of Auschwitz*, Exposition Press, New York.

Nietzsche, F 1980, *On the Advantage and Disadvantage of History for Life*, Hackett Books, New York.

Noakes, J & Pridham, G (eds) 1988, *Nazism: a History in Documents and Eyewitness Accounts 1919 – 1945*, Schocken Books, New York.

Nomberg-Przytyk, S, 1985, *Auschwitz: True Tales from a Grotesque Land*, University of North Carolina Press, Chapel Hill, NC.

Nyiszli, M 1993, *Auschwitz: A Doctor's Eyewitness Account*, Arcade Publishing, New York.

Ofer, D 2008, 'The Community and the Individual', in Bankier, D & Gutman, I (eds) 2003, *Nazi Europe and the Final Solution*, The Holocaust Martyrs' and Heroes' Remembrance Authority, Yad Vashem, Jerusalem.

Olbrycht, J 1945, testimony given at the trial of Rudolf Höss, Auschwitz-Birkenau State Museum Archives, *Collection Trial of Höss*, Vol. 59, Card 81.

Olère, D 1989, *The Eyes of a Witness*, Beate Klarsfeld Foundation, New York.

Olère, D & Oler, A 1998, *Witness: Images of Auschwitz*, Westwind Press, North Richland Hills, TX.

Padfield, P 2001, *Himmler: Reichsführer-SS*, Cassell & Co, London.

Pamięci, K 2002, *Transporty Polaków Do KL Auschwitz Z Krakowa: I Innych Miejscowości Polski Poludniowej 1940–1944*, vols 1–5, Towarzstwo Opieki Nad Oświęcim Państwowe Muzeum Auschwitz-Birkenau, Oświęcim.

PanstoPasternak, A 2006, *Inhuman Research: Medical Experiments in German Concentration Camps*, Akadémiai Kiadó, Budapest.

Park, CL Cohen, L & Murch, R 1996 Assessment and prediction of stress-related growth. Journal of Personality, 64, 71–105

Patai, R 1996, *The Jews of Hungary*, Wayne State University Press, Detroit, MI.

Pawelczyńska, A 1973, *Values and Violence in Auschwitz: a Sociological Analysis*, University of California Press, Berkeley, CA.

Pearlin, LL 2005, 'Some conceptual perspectives on the origins and prevention of social stress', in Maney, A & Ramos, J (eds) *Socioeconomic Conditions, Stress and Mental Disorders: toward a New Synthesis of Research and Public Policy*, National Institute of Mental Health, Washington, DC.

Pendas, DO 2006, *The Frankfurt Auschwitz Trial, 1963–1965: Genocide, History and the Limits of the Law*, Cambridge University Press, New York.

Perl, G 1984, *I Was a Doctor in Auschwitz*, Ayer Company Publishers Inc, North Stratford, NH.

Perl, G 1947, Letter from Perl to the Office of the US Chief of Counsel, War Department, Washington, DC, 11 January, accessed at US Holocaust Memorial Museum, courtesy of National Archives & Records Administration, Washington DC.

Perl, G 2004, *Out of the Ashes*. DVD. Directed by Joseph Sargent. Showtime Entertainment, USA.

Pervin, LA & John, OP (eds) 1999, *Handbook of Personality: Theory and Research* (2nd ed.), Guilford Press, New York.

Philips, R (ed) 1949, *Trial of Josef Kramer and Forty-Four Others (The Belsen Trial)*, William Hodge & Co, London.

Piper, F 2002, *Auschwitz Prisoner Labor*, Auschwitz-Birkenau State Museum, Oświęcim.

Piper, F & Świebocka, T (eds), 2000 *Auschwitz: Nazi Death Camp*, Auschwitz-Birkenau State Museum, Oświęcim.

Pogonowski, J 2000, *Illicit Letters from Auschwitz*, Frap Books, Oświęcim.

Poliakov, L 2003, *The History of Antisemitism: Suicidal Europe, 1870–1933*, vol. 4, University of Pennsylvania, Philadelphia, PA.

Poller, W 1971, *Medical Block Buchenwald: an Eyewitness Account of the Horrors of Buchenwald*, Corgi Books, London.

Prinz, J 2011, *Beyond Human Nature: How Culture and Experience Shape Our Lives*, Allen Lane, London.

Proctor, RN 1988, *Racial Hygiene: Medicine under the Nazis*, Harvard University Press, Cambridge, MA.

Pytell T 2000, 'The missing pieces of the puzzle: a reflection on the odd career of Viktor Frankl', *Journal of Contemporary History*, vol. 35, no. 2, pp. 281.

Rachman, S 1979. The concept of required helplessness. Behavioural Research and Therapy, 17, 1–6

Rees, L 2005, *Auschwitz: How Mankind Committed the Ultimate Infamy*, Public Affairs, New York.

Perl, G 2008, *Their Darkest Hour: People Tested to the Extreme in WWII*, Ebury Press, London.

Regehr, C Hill, J & Glancy, GD 2000 Individual predictors of traumatic in firefighters. Journal of Nervous and Mental Disease, 188, 333–339

Reich, J, Zautra, A & Hall JS (eds) 2010, *Handbook of Adult Resilience*, Guilford Press, New York.

Reinhold, N 1932, *Moral Man and Immoral Society*, Touchstone, New York.

Rittener, C & Myers, S 1986, *The Courage to Care*, New York University Press, New York.

Ritvo, RA & Plotkin, DM 1998, *Sisters in Sorrow: Voices of Care in the Holocaust*, Texas A & M University Press, College Station, TX.

Roland, CG 1992, *Courage Under Siege: Starvation, Disease and Death in the Warsaw Ghetto*, Oxford University Press, New York.

Roseman, M 2002, *The Villa, the Lake, the Meeting: Wannsee and the Final Solution*, Penguin, London.

Rosenstein, P 1954, *Narben bleiben zurück: die Lebenserrinerungen des großen jüdischen Chirurgen*, Kindler & Schiermeyer, München.

Rosenzweig, H 1948, Written testimony of, document 0-3/437, Yad Vashem Archives, Jerusalem.

Roth, JK & Maxwell, E 2001, *Remembering for the Future: The Holocaust in an Age of Genocide*, vol. 1, Palgrave, New York.

Rousset, D 1947, *The Other Kingdom*, Reynal & Hitchcock, New York.

Rubenfeld, S (ed) 2010, *Medicine after the Holocaust: from the Master Race to the Human Genome and Beyond*, Palgrave Macmillan, New York.

Rubenstein, RL & Roth, JK 2006, *Approaches to Auschwitz: The Holocaust and Its Legacy*, John Knox Press, Atlanta.

Rubin, A & Greenspan, H 2006, *Reflections: Auschwitz, Memory and a Life Recreated*, Paragon House, St Paul, MI.

Rutter, M 1997. Psychological resilience and protective mechanisms. American Journal of of Orthopsychiatry, 57,316–331.

Roth, JK 2007, *In the Shadow of Birkenau*, Palgrave MacMillan, Houndmills, Hampshire.

Schlesak, D 2001, *The Druggist of Auschwitz: A Documentary Novel*, Farrar, Straus & Giroux, New York.

Schnabel, R 1957, *Macht ohne Moral: eine Dokumentation über die SS*, Röderbergverlag, Frankfurt/Main.

Seemanova, A n.d., Written memoir of Dr Anna Seemanowa, File 4668, Jewish Historical Institute, Warsaw.

Seligman, MEP 2002, Authentic happiness. New York: Free Press

Sereny, G 2000, *The German Trauma: Experiences and Reflections 1938–2001*, Penguin, London.

Sereny, G 1974, *Into the Darkness*, McGraw-Hill, New York.

Setkiewicz, P 2008, *The Histories of Auschwitz IG Farben Werk Camps 1941–1945*, Auschwitz-Birkenau State Museum, Oświęcim.

Shakespeare, W 1963, *King Lear*, Methuen & Co, London.

Shantall, T 2002, *Life's Meaning in the Face of Suffering: Testimonies of Holocaust Survivors*, Magnes Press, Jerusalem.

Shavit, S & Michman, D 2009, 'How is a study of hell to be undertaken? Leni Yahil – 50 years of research into the Holocaust', *Yad Vashem Studies*, vol. 36 no.1, pp. 9.

Shelley, L 1991, *Criminal Experiments on Human Beings in Auschwitz and War Research Laboratories: Twenty Women Prisoners' Accounts*, Mellen Research University Press, San Francisco, CA.

Shelley, L 1986, *Secretaries of Death*, Shergold Publishers, New York.

Shelley, P 1907, *The Lyrics and Shorter Poems of Percy Bysshe Shelley*, JM Dent and Sons, London.

Shoah 1985, 2008 DVD, Umbrella Entertainment, Australia. Directed by Claude Lanzmann. Suedfeld, P 2003, 'Specific and general attributional patterns of Holocaust survivors', *Canadian Journal of Behavioural Science*, vol. 35, no. 2, pp. 133.

Skodol, AE 2010, 'The Resilient Personality' in Zautra, A & Hall, JS (eds), *Handbook of Adult Resilience*, Guilford Press, New York.

Smoleń, K (ed) 1976, *From the History of KL Auschwitz*, vol. 2, Państwowe Muzeum, Oświęcim.

Soet, JE Black GA & Dilorio , C 2003 Preference and predictors of women's experience of psychological experience of psychological trauma during child birth . Birth, 30, 36–46

Sofsky, W 1993, *The Order of Terror: The Concentration Camp*. Princeton University Press, Princeton, NJ.

Southwick, SM Vythilingam, M & Charney DS 2005. The psychobiology of depression ans resilience to stress: Implications for prevention and treatment. Annual Review of Clinical Psychology , 1, 255–291

Sperber, K 1946, Statement given to United Nations War Crimes Group June 1946, United States Holocaust Memorial Museum Archives, Washington, DC.

Stanescu, C & Morosanu, P 2005. Neoroticism, Ego, Defence Mechanisms & Valoric Types: a correlative study. Vol. 1, No. 1 Europe's Journal of Psychology

Spitz, V 2005, *Doctors from Hell: the Horrific Account of Nazi Experiments on Humans*, Sentient Publications, Boulder, CO.

Stanton, AL Parsa, A & Austenfeld, JL 2002. The adaptive potential of coping through emotional approach. In C.R. Snyder & S. J. Lopez (Eds.) Handbook of positive psychology (pp 148-158). New York: Oxford University Press

State Museum of Auschwitz-Birkenau (ed) 1995, *Death Books from Auschwitz: Remnants Reports*, KG Saur, München.

Staub, E 2003, *The Psychology of Good and Evil: Why Children, Adults and Groups Help and Harm Others*, Cambridge University Press, Cambridge.

Steinbacher, S 2005, *Auschwitz: A History*, Penguin, New York.

Stevenson, J (ed) 1985, *Recent Research in Developmental Psychopathology*, Elssford, Pergamon, NY.

Strzelecka, I 2008, *Voices of Memory 2: Medical Crimes, the Experiments in Auschwitz*, Auschwitz-Birkenau State Museum, Oświęcim.

Strzelecka, I 2008, *Voices of Memory 3: Medical Crimes, the Hospitals in Auschwitz*, Auschwitz-Birkenau State Museum, Oświęcim.

Suedfeld, P 2003, 'Specific and General Attributional Patterns of Holocaust Survivors', *Canadian Journal of Behavioural Science*, vol. 35, no. 2, pp. 133.

Świebocka, T (ed) 2001, *The Architecture of Crime: The 'Central Camp Sauna' in Auschwitz II-Birkenau*, Auschwitz-Birkenau State Museum, Oświęcim.

Szabó, É & Róder, L (eds) 1999, *In the Name of Humanity: Doctors and Medical Professionals Who Saved Lives in 1944–1945*, Association of Hungarian Resistance Fighters and Anti-Fascists and the VII/5 Branch of the Red Cross, Budapest.

Szende, S 1945, *The Promise Hitler Kept*, Victor Gollancz, London.

Szmaglewska, S 2001, *Smoke over Birkenau*, Książka i Wiedza, Warsaw.

Tatz, C 2001, *Genocide Perspectives I: Essays in Comparative Genocide*, Macquarie University, Sydney.

Taubenschlag, S 1998, *To Be a Jew in Occupied Poland*, Frap Books, Oświęcim.

Tec, N 2003, *Resilience and Courage: Women, Men and the Holocaust*, Yale University Press, New Haven, CT.

Tedeschi, G 1993, *There is a Place on Earth: a Woman in Birkenau*, Lime Tree, London.

Tedeschi, G Park, CL & Calhoun LG {Eds}. Posttraumatic growth: Positive changes in the aftermath of crisis. Mahwah NJ: Erlbaum

Tenenbaum, J 1963, 'The Jews in Poland', in Falstein, L (ed), *The Martyrdom of Jewish Doctors in Poland*, Exposition Press Inc, New York.

The Liberation of Auschwitz 1986, documentary, Artsmagic, United Kingdom, original release *Die Befreiung von Auschwitz*, Chronos, Germany. Directed by Ingrid von zur Mühlen.

United States Holocaust Memorial Museum (USHMM) 2012 Archives 1946, Recordings of Rudolph Höss Trial, vol. 22, Accessed at US Holocaust Memorial Museum, courtesy of National Archives & Records Administration, Washington DC.

United States Holocaust Memorial Museum (USHMM) Archives Excerpt from memoirs of Wieslaw Kielar, prisoner number 290, APMAB, Recollections Fond, Vol. 64, Accessed at US Holocaust Memorial Museum, courtesy of National Archives & Records Administration, Washington DC.

United States Holocaust Memorial Museum (USHMM) 2012 Archives Document No-205, Office of the U.S. Chief of Counsel, in RG-30.001M, Accessed at US Holocaust Memorial Museum, courtesy of National Archives & Records Administration, Washington DC.

United States Holocaust Memorial Museum (USHMM) 2012 Archives Memorandum on Conference, Document NO-216, RG-30.00M.

United States Holocaust Memorial Museum (USHMM) 2013 Archives List of Male Transports to Auschwitz. APMO, D-RO/123., vol. 20.

United States Holocaust Memorial Museum (USHMM) 2013 Archives List of Female Transports to Auschwitz. APMO, D-RO/123, vol. 20.

United States Holocaust Memorial Museum (USHMM) United States Holocaust Archives Richard Van Dam, Eyewitness Account, Doc.5, P. III h. N782 Auschwitz, Trials of War Criminals before the Nuremberg Military Tribunals, Washington 1950 Vol.5.

United States Holocaust Memorial Museum (USHMM) 2013 Archives Statement by Dr Karel Sperber, United Nations War Crimes Group, June 1946.

United States Holocaust Memorial Museum (USHMM) 2013 Archives Statement by Office of the US Chief Counsel, War Department, Washington D.C. January 11, 1947.

Unsdorfer, SB 1983, *The Yellow Star*, Feldheim Publishers, Jerusalem.

Uris, L 1958, *Exodus*, Doubleday, New York.

Vaillant, G 1992, *Ego Mechanisms of Defence: a Guide for Clinicians and Researchers*, American Psychiatric Press, Washington.

Vaillant, G 1993, *The Wisdom of the Ego*, Harvard University Press, Cambridge, MA.

Vaisman, S 2005, *A Jewish Doctor in Auschwitz: The Testimony of Sima Vaisman*, Melville House Publishing, Hoboken, NJ.

Valent, P 1998, 'Resilience in child survivors of the Holocaust: toward the concept of resilience', *Psychoanalytic Review*, vol. 85, no. 4, pp. 517.

Verdict on Auschwitz: The Frankfurt Auschwitz Trial 1963–1965 2005, DVD, Hessischer Rundfunk, Germany. Directed by Rolf Bickel & Dietrich Wagner.

Vitz, P & Mago P 1997, 'Kleinian psychodynamics and religious aspects of hatred as a defence mechanism', *Journal of Psychology and Theology*, vol. 25, no. 1, pp. 64.

Wagnon, BD 1976, 'Communication: the key element to prisoner of war survival', Air University Review, May-June, viewed 10 August 2014, www.airpower.maxwell.af.mil/airchronicles/aureview/1976/may-June/wagon.html

Wade, SL Borawski, EA Taylor, HG Drotar, D Yeates, KO & Stancin, T 2001. The relationship of caregiver coping to family outcomes during the initial year following pediatric traumatic injury. Journal of Consulting and Clinical Psychology, 69, 406-415

Waite, T 1993, *Taken on Trust: Collections from Captivity* Hodder & Stoughton, London.

Wajnryb, R 2002, *The Silence: How Tragedy Shapes Talk*, Allen and Unwin, Sydney.

Weikart, R 2004, *From Darwin to Hitler: Evolutionary Ethics, Eugenics and Racism in Germany*, Palgrave Macmillan, New York.

Weinberger, RJ 2009, *Fertility Experiments in Auschwitz-Birkenau: Perpetrators and Their Victims*, Südwestdeutscher Verlag, Saarbrücken.

Weindling, P 2000, *Epidemics and Genocide in Eastern* Europe *1890–1945*, Oxford University Press, Oxford.

Weiner, M 1999, *Jewish Roots in Ukraine and Moldova: Pages from the Past and Archival Inventories*, Miriam Weiner Roots to Roots Foundation, Secaucus, NJ.

Weiss, J 1996, *Ideology of Death: Why the Holocaust Happened in Germany*, Ivan R Dee, Chicago, IL.

Weiss, J 2003, *The Politics of Hate: Antisemitism, History and the Holocaust in Modern Europe*, Ivan R Dee, Chicago, IL.

Weiss, L 2003, *My Two Lives*, Sydney Jewish Museum, Sydney.

Weissman, G 2004, *Fantasies of Witnessing: Postwar Efforts to Experience the Holocaust*, Cornell University Press, London.

Werner, EE 1990 'High-risk children in young adulthood: longitudinal study from birth to 32 years' in Chess, S & Hertzig, ME (eds), *Annual Progress in Child Psychiatry and Child Development*, Brunner Mazel, Philadelphia.

Wiernicki, J 2001, *War in the Shadow of Auschwitz: Memoirs of a Polish Resistance Fighter and Survivor of the Death Camps*, Syracuse University Press, Syracuse, NY.

Wiesel, E 2006, *Night*, Penguin, London.

Wildt M 2000, 'Violence Against Jews in Germany, 1933–1939', in Bankier, D (ed), *Probing the Depth of German Antisemitism*, Yad Vashem, Jerusalem.

Winick, M (ed) 1997, *Hunger Disease: Studies by the Jewish Doctors in the Warsaw Ghetto*, vol. 7, John Wiley & Sons, New York.

Wittmann, R 2005, *Beyond Justice: the Auschwitz Trial*, Harvard University Press, Cambridge, MA.

Wolfgang, S 1997, *The Order of Terror: the Concentration* Camp, Princeton University Press, Princeton, NJ.

Yad Vashem Archives, Jerusalem. 2012 Conference of Heydrich's division heads and Einsatz-gruppen, September 21, 1939. NA Microfilm, T175/239/2728524-28.

Yahil, L 1990, *The Holocaust: the Fate of European Jewry*, Oxford University Press, NY.

Zautra, A, Hall, JS & Murray, K 2010, 'Resilience: A New Definition of Health for People and Communities' in Zautra, A & Hall, JS (eds), *Handbook of Adult Resilience*, Guilford Press, New York.

Zelizer, B 1998, *Remembering to Forget: Holocaust Memory through the Camera's Eye*, Chicago University Press, Chicago, IL.

Zywulska, K 2009, *I Survived Auschwitz*, Auschwitz-Birkenau State Museum, Oświęcim.

Glossary

Abteilung V	Camp medical centre
Aktions	This word was a euphemism for the group killing of Jews or gypsies after a selection in the camps or after rounding up Jews in towns in Nazi controlled territory
Arbeitslager	Labor camp
Arbeit Macht Frei	Work will make you free
Ärtz	Doctor
Ärztlicher Bericht	Medical records
Auschwitz I	Main camp
Auschwitz II	Birkenhau – Labor camp
Auschwitz III	Monowitz – Industrial camp
Brezinka	Birkenhau
Block 10	Experimental block
Block 11	Punishment block
Block 19	Surgery block – part of experiment operations
Blockälteste	Senior block prisoner
Blockarzt	Block prisoner doctor
Blockova	Prisoner in charge of a block
Blockschreiber	Prisoner block clerk
DP	Displaced Persons
Defense Mechanism	Conscience and un-conscience actions and behaviour providing prisoners with protection and respite
Drancy	Transit camp
Durchfall	Diarrhea
Durchgangsjuden	Jews in transit not recorded in Auschwitz arrival registry. Murdered upon arrival.
Einsatzgruppen	Mobile forces of the Security Police and SS Security Service that followed the German armies through Eastern Europe killing all Jewish inhabitants
Geheimnisträeger	Keeper of secrets
Ghetto	In Nazi occupied territories Jews were confined to tightly packed areas within a city precinct
Generalgouvernement	Nazi Political administrative centre of Poland
Glinka biala	White clay
Hauptsturmführer	Rank of Captain
Hekdesh	a ghetto hospital, refuge for the sick, the destitute and the old
Himmelkommando	Workgroup in the sky – reference to prisoners sent to the gas chambers and then ovens
Hygiene Institute of the Waffen-SS in Raisko	Institute of research located approximately five kilometres from the main camp
JDC	Joint Distribution Committee
Kanada	Collection centre of possessions brought to Auschwitz by Jews
Kapo	A prisoner assigned by the SS to supervise forced labor or carry out administrative tasks

https://doi.org/10.1515/9783110598216-021

Krankenbehändler	Sick treaters
Krankenhaus	Hospital
Krankenlager	Hospital camp
Krankenrevier	Medical blocks in which patients after selections were kept before sent to be gassed
Lagerarzt	Camp doctor
Mechelen	Transit camp
Medizinischer Dienst der KL	Medical service for concentration camps
Mikva	ritual bath
Monowitz concentration camp	Auschwitz III
Muselmänner	was a slang term used to refer to those suffering from a combination of starvation and exhaustion resigned to their impending death.
Neirentzündung	Fatal injection
Neustadt-Glewe	Concentration camp
Non nocere	Do no harm
numerus clausus	one of many methods used to limit the number of students who may study at a university
Noma	A gangrenous disease leading to tissue destruction of the face, particularly the mouth and face.
Oberschwester	Head Nurse
Organizing	Stealing
Philosemites	Respect for and an appreciation of Jewish people, their history and the influence of Judaism, particularly on the part of a gentile.
POW	Prisoner of War
Ramp	Area of arrival of trains at which selections took place deciding who would be gassed and who would go to the labor camps
Ravensbrück	Concentration camp
Revier	Hospital ward
Schreibstube	Administration office
Selections	Condemning prisoners unable to work to death
Sonderbehandlung	Special treatment sending prisoners to the gas
Sonderkommando	Prisoners (mainly Jewish) selected to work in the crematorium placing the dead into the ovens and then cleaning the ovens of human ash
Stammlager	Auschwitz I, Main camp
SS-Standortarzt	Chief garrison SS physician
Tanakh	Term used for the Hebrew scriptures
Theresienstadt	Concentration camp and ghetto
Tisanes	Gypsies
Totenbuch	Death book
Totenmeldungen	Death certificate
Untersturmführer	Second Lieutenant

Appendices I

Report by Dr. Kurt Grunwald
(Czechslov. physician)

Prague II, Vojtasaha 11
At present:
Stadtilm, Marktplatz 34

    In September 1938 I sent my wife and our two boys to
Jugoslavia and I led in accordance with my mobilisation order
as first-lieutenant the surgical department of the military
hospital in Bratislava. At the end of November I have been
demobilized, met my family in Prague and as the danger of
Nazi invasion became imminent I decided to emigrate and applied in December 1938 for immigration to the U.S. Although
I have a brother-in-law, an American citizen, in New ... ,
my hopes were frustrated by the German authorities, who
after the occupation on 15 March 1939 did not allow me to
leave the country. On July 13, 1942 they seized that remained
of my already partly robbed property and brought me with my
family to the "Ghetto" Terezin (Theresienstadt) near Lito-
merice (Leitmeritz). There was crammed into the old fortress
destined for 4000 inhabitants a population of 70-80,000 jewish
families from all over Europe. The conditions were bad.
Before putting us in, all facilities, the ramshackle buildings
could offer had been removed. There was not a single chair
to sit on, nor a table to eat by, nor a single bed. I slept
on the floor of a dirty former butcher shop for 3 weeks,
then I was put in a barrack for ten where the inhabitants
slept in wooded beds of mostly three decks. My wife slept
for one and a half years on the floor. The number of fleas,
bugs and lice reached astronomical heights. All previous
things, jewels, watches, money, fountain-pens, paper (including toilet-paper), candles, matches and all valuable food
had been taken from us on our arrival. There was an epidemic
of dysentorie, people died by the hundreds a day. The buildings became stinking pestholes. It was forbidden to communicate with the outer world. Six months before our arrival
18 young men had been publicly hung because they had written
to their mothers that they were suffering from hunger. When
we came to Terezin letter writing was still forbidden under
death penalty. Whoever did not greet a German was punished
with 20 blows with a stick. Smoking was punished with imprisonment for two weeks. Every day there arrived new transports for the most part of czechoslovakien, german, austrian
and netherland jews. On the other side, transports were
sent from Terezin to the "East". As we later understood,
these transports went for the most part to "Birkenau"
(Auschwitz) to be gased and burned.
    On December 15, 1943 I was sent with my family into this
greatest camp of extermination. For 6 months I worked there
as physician in the same camp where my wife...
On March 6, 1944 were taken 3800 persons...
healthy people with 600 children among them... gased and burned
during one night.

Incl. No. 2

Grunwald Testimony

Dr. Kurt Grunwald's testimony of he and his families captivity and fate in Auschwitz

https://doi.org/10.1515/9783110598216-022

Page 2 Grunwald

'CONFIDENTI '

During May and June I saw daily the arrival of 10 to
20,000 hungarian and carpatorumian jewish families of whom
at least 80% were immediately gassed and burned. Day and
night 4 crematories were blyzing, they did not suffice.
The corpses had to be burned in large holes nearby. The
smoke and the stink of burned flesh and bones went straight
into our barracks. I have been told that occasionally
women and children have been thrown alive into the flames.
I did not see such things, but I heard during several nights
loud cries and crying children, cries which meant utter
death anxiety, barking of dogs, rifle and machine-gun fire.
During the first months of 1944 I assisted 14 women in
childbirth. There were born 13 healthy children. The SS
physician showed himself interested in the welfare of
mothers and children. They were exceptionally well fed,
they received milk, fresh butter and pudding. On july 10
and 11 all women with their children , all old and rich have
been gased and burned. Among these also my young and healthy
wife, Wilma, my son John and my 71 year old mother who as
still in good health. My 11 year old son Michael, who was a
good-looking little fellow with fair hair and blue eyes (as
the Germans like it) has been spared and got into another
camp. After this catastrophe I worked as physician in the
hospital camp adjoining the four crematories. I was present
at a great number of selections where thousands of weak and
sick have been gased and burned. My little boy came once
a week to see me.
On October 26, 1944 happened what I feared most—I was
separated from my boy. I was sent with a transport of labourers to Ohrdruf and my boy stayed in Birkenau. Members
of the SS told me, that there wasn't any danger for my son.
I know what value there is in nazi promises and I hope only
that my boy has been liberated by the russians when they
entered Auschwitz in January.
In Ohrdruf I worked for two weeks in the rocks, afterwards as physician. Ohrdruf was a cold crematorium. People
of all nations; Russians, Poles, Hungarians, Yougoslaves,
Czechs, Italiens and French were murdered by hard labour
without appropriate clothing and food, the lack of sleep and
rest and by the lice. At last by beating within an inch of
their lives or by beating to death. When the order of evacuation came on April 3rd, it never entered our mind that
they could move 20,00 sick, among these many with typhus
and high fever. But they drove all on the road and drove us
physicians with them during the whole night to Arnstadt,
and during the following day over Stadtilm in the direction
of Rudolstadt. Who could not follow had been abandoned on
the road. Many are said to have been shot. I have not
seen it. There are rumours that numbers of evacuated prisoners have been buried in nearby villages. These things
should be investigated, and if true, the corpses exhumated
and if possible indentified. On the fourth of April before
nightfall we persuaded the guards to stay for the night in
a barn near Ehrnstein. At dawn I escaped with my french
colleague Dr. Gabay in the forest. We stayed in the forest
eight days, mostly in the midst of the american CANCELLED
artillery fire and were saved by the american army in the
evening of April 12th.

CONFIDENTIAL

Joseph W...... ......, Major, A.C.
.....da Center
7708 War Crimes Group, 1 March 1948

Inel No. 2

USHMM

The report by Dr. Kurt Grunwald details his and his families' experiences and fate in the
SS ghettoes and concentration camps from 1939 to 1945.

Appendice II

Telegram from Heinrich Schwarz, prisoner labor chief in KL Auschwitz, to Department D II of the WVHA, dated February 20, 1943, concerning 5,022 Jews deported in three transports from the Theresienstadt ghetto, including information on the totals and percentages of people selected for work or gassed (*Sonderunterbringung*, separate placement)

Dr Wolkens' source of information (telegram) of prisoner arrivals to Auschwitz

Appendices 7.1

Auschwitz-Birkenau
w Oświęcimiu -
DZIAŁ ARCHIWUM

Załącznik Nr. 6b.
/str. 11 protokołu/
114

Kommentar zu den Statistiken I und II.
betreffend 15 Juden-Transporte, die in der Zeit vom 17.IV.1942 bis 17.VII.1942 in das Konzentrationslager Auschwitz aufgenommen wurden.

Die vorliegenden beiden Statistiken behandeln das Schicksal derjenigen Juden, die das scheinbare Glueck hatten, nach ihrer Ankunft in Auschwitz nicht sofort ins Gas geschickt, sondern ins Lager aufgenommen zu werden. Dieses Glueck erwies sich bald als truegerisch, denn ihr Ziel - der Tod war dasselbe, nur der Weg dahin unsagbar schwer unter vielen Martern und Qualen, blutgetraenkt. Grundlage dieser Statistiken bildet ein in Auschwitz voegefundenes Originalfascikel, das den Titel fuehrt, "Zugangslisten Juden, nicht fotografiert". Diese Mappe umfasst die Zugangslisten von 15 juedischen Transporten, jede Liste enthalten Haeftlingsnummer, Name, Vorname, Geburtsort und Datum und Beruf. Neben den Familiennamen, oder Vornamen - je nach Platz - ist mit Bleistift das jeweilige Todesdatum eingetragen.

In der Statistik I sind diese 15 Transporte nach dem Kalenderdatum erfasst und fuer jeden Tag aus jedem der einzelnen Transporte die Totenziffer eingetragen. Das Zugangsdatum des Transportes ist durch einen schwarzen wagrechten Strich gekennzeichnet. Das Schicksal der einzelnen Transporte sieht wie folgt aus. Leider wurde mit dem 15.6.1942 aufgehoert das Todesdatum einzusetzen, so dass wir fuer die nachfolgende Zeit nur Schluesse aus den anderen Transporten ziehen koennen.

Transport I, zugegangen am 15.IV.1942 aus der Slovakei, umfassend 973 Haeftlinge. Am vorerwaehnten Stichtag, den 15.August 42, waren von ihnen 665 getoetet und nur mehr 88 ... am Leben.

Transport II, zugegangen am 19.IV.1942 aus der Slovakei, umfassend 464 Haeftlinge, Am Stichtag lebten von ihnen nur sehr 10 ...

Report by Wolken regarding the fate of the prisoners after arrival

Appendices 7.2

ji.   - 2 -   **115**

Transport III, zugegangen am 22.IV.1942 aus der Slovakei, umfassend 543 Haeftlinge, am Stichtag lebten 41 = 7.5%.

Transport IV, zugegangen am 27.IV.1942 aus der Slovakei, umfassend 442 Haeftlinge, am Stichtag lebten 23 = 5-2%.

Transport V, zugegangen am 29.IV.1942 aus der Slovakei, umfassend 423 Haeftlinge, am Stichtag lebten 20 = 4-7%.

Transport VI, zugegangen am 22.V.1942, ueberstellt aus dem K.L. Lublin, slovakische Juden 1000, am Stichtag lebten 52 = 5.3%.

Transport VII, zugegangen am 7.VI.1942, eingeliefert vom Reichssicherheitsamt / R.S.H.A./ aus Paris, umfassend Juden aller Nationalitaeten, 1000, am Stichtag lebten 217 = 21.7%.

Transprt VIII, zugegangen am 20.VI.1942 aus der Slovakei, umfassend 404 Haeftlinge, am Stichtag lebten 45 = 11.1%.

Transport IX, zugegangen am 24.VI.1942, eingeliefert vom R.S.H.A. aus Paris, umfassend Juden aller Nationalitaeten, 933, am Stichtag lebten 186 = 20%.

Transport X, zugegangen am 27.VI.1942, eingeliefert vom R.S.H.A. Polnische Juden, 1000, am Stichtag lebten 557 = 55.7%.

Transport XI, zugegangen am 30.VI.1942, eingeliefert vom R.S.H.A. Polnische Juden, 1004, am Stichtag lebten 703 = 70%.

Transport XII, zugegangen am 30.VI.1942, ueberstellt aus dem K.L. Lublin, Slovakische Juden 400 es lebten am Stichtag 208 = 52%.

Transport XIII, zugegangen am 4.VII.1942, eingeliefert vom R.S.H.A. Slovakische Juden, 264, es lebten am Stichtag 69 = 30%.

Transport XIV, zugegangen am 11.VII.1942 aus der Slovakei, umfassend, 182 Haeftlinge, am Stichtag lebten 64 = 35%.

Transport XV, zugegangen am 17.VII.1942, eingeliefert vom R.S.H.A. Hollaendische Juden, 651, am Stichtag lebten 426 = 30%.

Die 15 Transporte umfassen insgesamt 9853 Haeftlinge, von denen 6973 bis 15.8.42 getoetet waren, dass es nicht dabei um willkuerliche Toetungsaktionen handelte, ergibt sich aus der geben

Appendices 7.3

ueberstellung der Totenziffern an verschiedenen Tagen. So gab es
beispielsweise am 16 Juni 42 aus den schon zu dieser Zeit im Lager befindlichen 7 Transporten 41 Tote, am 17 Juni - dem Tage des
Besuches Himmlers im Lager - gab es ueberhaupt keine Toten. Dafuer
wurde am naechsten Tage, dem 18.6., dieses Manko mit einer Toten-
zahl von 80 aufgeholt. Es ist bei Betrachtung der Statistiken der
Gedanke nicht von der Hand zu weisen, dass damals spezielle Auf-
traege zur raschen Toetung der Menschen gegeben wurden, denn waeh-
rend sich bis zu dieser Zeit die Totenzahlen im allgemeinen zwi-
schen 20 - 40 bewegten, stiegen sie von diesem Zeitpunkt an rapid
auf, so dass wir am 18.6.42 - 80, am 19.6. - 146 Tote zaehlen.
Der 20.Juni war scheinbar wieder ein Feiertag, denn an diesem Tage
gibt es nur 4 Tote. Am 21.6. - 89, am 22.6. - 104,und so bewegen
sich diese Totenzahlen von nun an weiter, die Tage mit den hoech-
sten Totenzahlen sind der 25.7.mit 162, der 28.7.mit 169,der 10.8.
mit 166 und der 12.8.mit 159 Toten.

Wenn wir die einzelnen Transporte vom nationalen Stand -
punkt aus betrachten, so faellt es auf,dass die Transporte der
Hollandischen und Slovakischen Juden eine viel rascher gehende
Vernichtung aufweisen, als die Transporte der Polnischen Juden,
die sich im allgemeinen gut hielten.

Am Fusse der Statistik I ergibt die erste wagrechte
Zahlenkolonne die Anzahl der Getoeteten aus jedem Transport, die
zweite Kolonne die Zahl der ueberhaupt mit jedem Transport Zugegangen, die dritte Zahlenkolonne die Zahl der am 15.August 1942
noch Lebenden. Wenn bei einzelnen Transporten diese Ziffer eine
scheinbar hohe ist, so muss darauf Ruecksicht genommen werden,
dass es soch um Transporte handelt, die sich nur verhaeltnismaes-
sog kurze Zeit im Lager aufgehalten haben.

Um nun ein klares Bild darueber zu bekommen, fuer wie-

Index

https://doi.org/10.1515/9783110598216-023